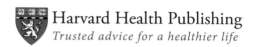
Harvard Health Publishing
Trusted advice for a healthier life

MW00720825

Dear Reader,

For a disease that affects more than 54 million adults in the United States—approximately one in five—arthritis is remarkably misunderstood. Arthritis is not a single disease. In fact, there are more than 100 different types of arthritis. Though all of them affect joints, their causes and treatments can vary considerably.

This report focuses primarily on osteoarthritis, which is the most common type of arthritis, affecting over 30 million Americans. Despite a solid body of knowledge about osteoarthritis, myths abound. For example, symptoms are not caused by changes in the weather, and people don't develop arthritis from being under too much stress, having allergies, or cracking their knuckles too much. And unless you are a jackhammer operator or a serious athlete prone to high-impact injuries, you are unlikely to develop it from overusing your joints.

Nor is osteoarthritis an inevitable part of growing old. Plenty of people age well without much arthritis—and for those that do develop it, there are now better treatments, so the disease doesn't have to be severely disabling.

In this report, you'll learn how osteoarthritis affects joints and how it is diagnosed. Because describing your symptoms is so important for a correct diagnosis, this report discusses the variety of symptoms that may occur. Equally important, you'll learn about treatment. While osteoarthritis is painful and can interfere with your ability to do things you enjoy, there are many steps you can take to protect your joints, reduce discomfort, and improve mobility. This report includes information on established medical therapies as well as complementary treatments such as acupuncture, chiropractic care, and massage. Because living with osteoarthritis requires more than taking pills, a Special Section provides advice about how to care for yourself through exercise, diet, and useful gadgets that make it easier to grasp items, open jars, and perform a host of daily activities.

Though treatment usually centers on managing the pain, researchers are examining possible new treatments that might halt or even reverse the effects of osteoarthritis. These are discussed in the report as well.

Millions of people must live with arthritis. This report suggests ways to live well.

Sincerely,

Robert H. Shmerling, M.D.
Medical Editor

Harvard Health Publishing | Harvard Medical School | 4 Blackfan Circle, 4th Floor | Boston, MA 02115

Your joints

If you have achy knees, hips, fingers, ankles, shoulders, or other joints, you are in good company. Many people have joint pain, and arthritis is a common cause. The word arthritis is derived from the Greek word *arthron* (joint) and the suffix *-itis* (inflammation), and it refers to any of roughly 100 diseases affecting the joints—including osteoarthritis, rheumatoid arthritis, gout, pseudogout, ankylosing spondylitis, and psoriatic arthritis. For people who have any of these forms of arthritis, the word variously signifies the pain, swelling, and stiffness that may be caused by tissue injury or disease in the joint. Together, all of the arthritic conditions are referred to as rheumatic diseases, and doctors who specialize in treating them are called rheumatologists. (The term rheumatism refers broadly to connective tissue disorders that cause pain and stiffness.)

Osteoarthritis, the most common type of arthritis, is a degenerative joint disease that results from the deterioration of the cartilage in the joints. It affects nearly half of Americans over age 65 and is the main focus of this report. But before examining the specific changes that occur in osteoarthritis—and the treatments that can help relieve arthritis pain—it's useful to understand the anatomy of joints and how they function. The terms defined in the next section, such as cartilage and synovium, will be used throughout the report.

Joint anatomy and function

The musculoskeletal system—that is, your muscles, bones, and connective tissues—could not be a more practical system for supporting your body, enabling movement, and protecting vital organs, like the heart, lungs, and brain.

A model of a skeleton may look rickety and frail, but bones have a compression strength equaling that of cast iron or oak. Although incredibly light—the average adult skeleton weighs only 20 pounds or so—bones are capable of bearing a tremendous load. Their strength is necessary to withstand potentially lethal blows to key organs and manage the more mundane forces of movement. When you walk at a leisurely pace, for example, each foot strikes the ground with a force about three times your weight. At a brisk walk or run, the pressure increases to five to six times your weight. In other words, a 150-pound person's lower extremities are repeatedly subjected to 450 to 900 pounds of force during normal daily activity.

These and other movements would not be possible without your joints—the places in the body where bones meet. Bones are held together at joints by tough bands of connective tissue called ligaments. Muscles then tug on bones to make them move, using the assistance of tendons, which attach the muscles to bones. Together, these structures stabilize the body, while allowing a remarkable variety of movement. But not all joints are alike.

Types of joints

The body contains three basic types of joints (see Figure 1, page 3), but not all of them develop arthritis.

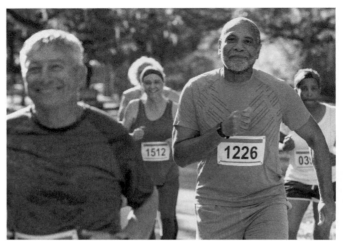

You have multiple types of joints. But synovial joints—those that enable most types of movement—are the ones most likely to develop osteoarthritis and cause pain and stiffness.

© kali9 | Getty Images

Fixed joints, or sutures, are thin bands of fibrous tissue that connect the platelike bones of the skull, allowing the skull to expand and accommodate the growing brain. When brain growth is complete, these fibrous joints disappear as the skull bones fuse. Osteoarthritis does not develop at fixed joints.

Cartilaginous joints contain tough cartilage plates. In the pelvis, these joints permit slight movement of the pubic bones. The discs between the vertebral bones in the spine are also cartilaginous joints. They are thick and accommodate mobility. The joints where the ribs meet the breastbone are also cartilaginous joints. Osteoarthritis can affect cartilaginous joints, but they are less susceptible to damage than synovial joints.

Synovial joints are the most mobile and the most susceptible to osteoarthritis. These are found in the shoulders, elbows, wrists, fingers, hips, knees, ankles, and toes. Synovial joints have a protective layer of cartilage covering the ends of the bones. But they take their name from the synovium, a membrane that lines the joint. The synovium produces synovial fluid, which provides nourishment and lubrication for the joints and allows them to be more mobile than cartilaginous joints. Synovial joints are designed for a variety of movements that make possible all manner of activity, from playing tennis to playing piano. Some—for example, the outermost joints of the fingers—are limited to flexion and extension (bending and straightening) within a single plane. Others, such as the shoulder, wrist, and hip, are capable of complex movements in multiple planes.

Built-in protection of synovial joints

Synovial joints, like machines with moving parts, are vulnerable to friction. If a machine's moving parts come in contact with one another, friction will scratch the surfaces and cause pitting, distortion, and eventually breakage. Two strategies can prevent such friction: applying a lubricant or inserting a cushion, such as a rubber gasket. Synovial joints are protected in both ways (see Figure 2, page 4). Following are the structures that help:

Synovial fluid. Lubrication comes from synovial fluid, a viscous, yellowish, translucent liquid that's produced by the synovium. This fluid not only oils the joint and minimizes friction; it also helps protect joints by forming a sticky seal that enables abutting bones to slide freely against each other, yet resist pulling apart. Synovial fluid also delivers vital nutrients, such as glucose, to the joint. This is an important function because cartilage does not have a blood supply. The thick consistency of synovial fluid comes in part from a substance called hyaluronic acid, which is also found in articular cartilage.

Figure 1: Types of joints

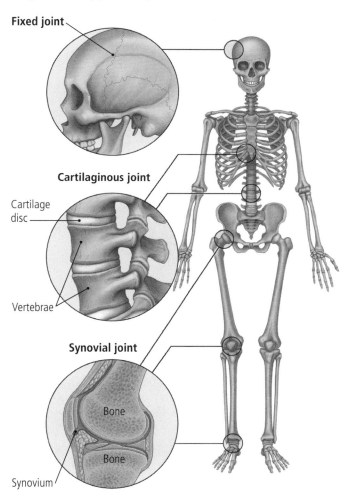

Fixed joint

Cartilaginous joint

Cartilage disc

Vertebrae

Synovial joint

Bone

Bone

Synovium

There are three basic types of joints. Fixed joints connect the platelike bones of the skull. Cartilaginous joints, such as those in the spine, contain tough plate-shaped structures that absorb shock and allow slight motion. The most mobile are synovial joints, which are surrounded by a loose fibrous capsule lined with a thin membrane called the synovium. These are most susceptible to osteoarthritis.

Articular cartilage. Cushioning is provided by articular cartilage, a tough and somewhat elastic tissue that covers the ends of bones. Because it's about 75% water, cartilage compresses under pressure (as occurs with jumping or even walking) and resumes its original thickness when the force is released, much like a very tough sponge. Because the articular cartilage can mold to its surroundings, the opposing surfaces of a joint are perfectly matched.

Figure 2: Anatomy of a synovial joint

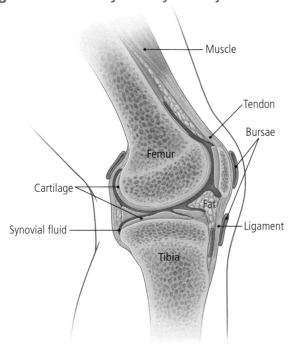

In a synovial joint such as the knee, shown here, ligaments bind the bones together and keep them in proper alignment. Muscles and their tendons stabilize the joint as well as move it. Cartilage, a tough and somewhat elastic tissue, provides a smooth, slippery surface for movement and cushions the joint. The viscous synovial fluid nourishes and lubricates the joint to provide nearly frictionless movement; it's produced by microscopic cells in the synovium, the membrane that lines the joint. The bursae allow the soft tissues around the joint to move smoothly as the joint moves.

Bursae. It's not just the inside surfaces of joints that are susceptible to damage. Places where tendons and muscles cross over a bone or another muscle are also subject to friction. These sites are protected by bursae, sacs that not only contain lubricating fluid but also act as cushions.

Stability in synovial joints

Several things help maintain stability through a joint's range of motion so that the joint can function normally. One is the contour and fit of the joint surfaces themselves. The hip, for example, is a ball-and-socket arrangement. With each stride, the head of the femur (thighbone) pushes deep into the cup-shaped cavity of the pelvis, providing maximum stability during walking. Most other joints, by contrast, are more like hinges.

Two forms of connective tissue—ligaments and tendons—also play an important role in joint structure and function. The main proteins that make up these tissues are collagens and elastins, which imbue them with tensile strength and elasticity.

Ligaments. Ligaments—the tough, slightly elastic, fibrous bands that bind one bone to another—also help with alignment. For example, ligaments on the sides of the finger joints prevent side-to-side bending, while ligaments stretching across the palm keep the fingers from bending too far backward.

Tendons. These are the fibrous cords that attach muscle to bone. Together with muscles, they stabilize joints as well as move them. The best example of how this works is in the shoulder, which has a wide range of motion that ligaments would impede. While the large, visible shoulder muscles supply the power to move the shoulder, the small rotator cuff muscles and tendons keep the head of the humerus (upper arm bone) from slipping out of the glenoid fossa, a shallow cuplike indentation in the shoulder blade. ♥

A closer look at osteoarthritis

Osteoarthritis develops when cartilage deteriorates. Over time, the space between bones narrows and the surfaces of the bones change shape, leading eventually to friction and joint damage. Osteoarthritis often affects more than one joint, and while it can strike almost any joint in the body, some are much more likely to be involved than others. For example, osteoarthritis is common in the hip, knee, lower back, neck, feet, and certain finger joints, but it is rare in the elbow.

The most common of all joint diseases, osteoarthritis affects over 30 million Americans. But this number only hints at the impact of osteoarthritis, which can send people to doctors' offices and pain clinics, make them reach for medications, keep them home from work, and curtail leisure and everyday activities. Women are more likely to have osteoarthritis than men, especially after age 50. While men tend to develop it most often in the hips, knees, and spine, women have it most often in the hands and knees—and they're 10 times more likely to develop Heberden's nodes (hard, bony growths that form on the joint nearest the fingertip). Genetics plays some role. People who have family members with osteoarthritis are more likely to develop osteoarthritis.

More than simple wear and tear

Osteoarthritis was long considered a natural product of aging, reflecting everyday wear and tear on cartilage. The demographics seemed to bear that out. The ailment is virtually unheard of in children and is rare in young adults, but common among older people and those who are overweight or obese.

Although wearing down of cartilage over time may be a factor, experts now believe the cause is likely more complex. External factors, such as injuries, are important initiators, and the rate of progression is probably affected by genes as well.

So how does osteoarthritis develop? The first signs are microscopic pits and fissures in the surface of the cartilage in your joints (see Figure 3, below). These fissures indicate that biochemical changes are gradually making the cartilage less resilient. Cartilage cells themselves produce enzymes that damage the molecules making up the structure of the cartilage, and tiny pieces of cartilage may flake off into the joint cavity. As a result, the shape of the cartilage lining the bone changes, leading to further damage as the deformed surfaces of articular cartilage move against each other.

Unfortunately, because cartilage lacks a blood supply, it has a limited ability to heal. As it degenerates, the ends of the two bones in a joint start to rub against each other. Just as a damaged gasket leads to metal-

Figure 3: Joint changes in osteoarthritis

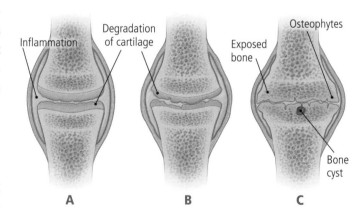

A. The first signs of osteoarthritis are microscopic pits and fissures on the cartilage surface, which are sometimes accompanied by inflammation.

B. The contours of the joint change, and the cartilage thins.

C. The bone surface thickens and osteophytes (abnormal bony growths) develop over time. Cartilage continues to wear away. The joint space narrows until it nearly disappears, leaving bone rubbing against bone. Bone cysts (open spaces filled with fluid) can develop as a reaction to stress on the bone.

on-metal contact in a machine, your bones experience mechanical friction and irritation. They try to repair themselves. But the renovation attempts are uneven, causing bony overgrowths, known as osteophytes, to form along the margins of the damaged joints. Bone cysts can also develop at the joint as a reaction to abnormal stress on bones. These cysts do not always cause symptoms, but they are noticeable on x-rays and are a sign of osteoarthritis.

Once your cartilage is damaged, the resulting abnormalities can irritate the surrounding soft tissues and cause inflammation. Doctors sometimes refer to osteoarthritis as noninflammatory to distinguish it from rheumatoid arthritis and other joint diseases in which inflammation is a cardinal feature. However, low-grade inflammation, with swelling and pain, is not unusual in osteoarthritis. People with severely damaged joints can also have episodes of synovitis (inflammation of the synovium, the lining of the joint). This inflammation tends to be milder than in rheumatoid arthritis. The combination of damaged cartilage, bone rubbing on bone, and inflammation makes movement painful.

Risk factors for osteoarthritis

Doctors sometimes categorize osteoarthritis as primary or secondary. In primary osteoarthritis, the principal cause is unknown, although age, excess weight, and genetics probably contribute. In secondary osteoarthritis, the disease originates from a significant injury (such as a fracture near a joint), past inflammation (from rheumatoid arthritis, for example), or a disorder such as hemophilia.

Primary osteoarthritis
While the exact reason cartilage deteriorates remains

▶ **Symptoms of osteoarthritis**
- Increased joint pain and swelling after activity
- Brief joint stiffness in the morning
- Grinding sensation when the joint is used
- Additional symptoms specific to the affected joint

a mystery, several factors are known to increase the likelihood of osteoarthritis.

Age. Degeneration of cartilage in joints occurs partly as a function of aging. But not everyone develops osteoarthritis. And, among those who do, the severity varies.

Excess weight. Being overweight or obese can lead to a host of health problems, including osteoarthritis. Weight-bearing joints such as the hips and knees are susceptible. For example, every additional pound of weight puts three to four pounds of pressure on the knee joint. Your knees simply don't hold up well under the continued strain of those extra pounds—and extra pounding.

One study found that obese women had about four times greater risk for knee osteoarthritis than non-obese women, and for obese men the risk was five times greater. An ongoing study of people living in Framingham, Mass., found that adults who were overweight in their 30s and 40s were more likely than their slimmer counterparts to develop osteoarthritis of the knee later in life. Women who were the heaviest were twice as likely as thinner women to get osteoarthritis—and when they did get it, they were more likely to develop a severe case. The heaviest women had three times the risk for severe knee osteoarthritis as the thinner ones. According to the CDC, close to 40% of adults in the United States are obese. Given the strong link between obesity and osteoarthritis, it is likely that the prevalence of knee osteoarthritis will continue to rise in this country.

Losing excess weight can greatly relieve pressure on joints, reducing the risk of developing osteoarthritis or, for people who already have the ailment, making daily living much easier. The Framingham study revealed that overweight women who lost an average of 11 pounds cut their risk of developing osteoarthritis of the knee by half.

Genetic factors. Most experts agree that genetic factors probably control the development and progression of osteoarthritis. Studies in identical twins—who share the same genes and thus offer insight into the relative importance of genetic and environmental factors—suggest that roughly half the risk of developing osteoarthritis can be attributed to genetic factors.

However, sorting out the contribution of various genes is not easy. Multiple genes are thought to play a role, and to complicate matters, these genes may have different effects depending on the joint in question and whether you're male or female.

Several factors limit genetic studies of a disease like osteoarthritis. First, the sheer number of people with the disorder makes it impossible to discount the influence of external factors. Second, scientists must establish that a certain gene is present in most people with the disease, but is absent in those who are healthy.

Secondary osteoarthritis

While the principal cause of primary arthritis is unknown, secondary osteoarthritis has a clear trigger, such as a significant injury or another disease.

Joint injury. As athletes know, severe knee injury disrupts the normal mechanics of joint function. Nearly all tissues heal by scarring, leaving irregularities on their surfaces. Because bones, joints, or muscles that are damaged rarely heal perfectly, joint injuries can create unusual mechanical stresses that lead to abnormal wear. Over time, this can result in osteoarthritis. In particular, a bone fracture near or through a joint is likely to cause cartilage deterioration and osteoarthritis.

While primary osteoarthritis is uncommon in the ankle, people who have had multiple serious ankle sprains or a fractured ankle can be at increased risk for developing secondary ankle osteoarthritis. Similarly, shoulder joints tend to hold up well against primary osteoarthritis. However, damage to other structures in the shoulder, such as the rotator cuff (four muscles and their tendons that surround and support the shoulder joint), can lead to osteoarthritis in the shoulder joint. The rotator cuff can tear suddenly from an injury or fray over time, leading to a tear.

People in certain occupations that put excessive stress on joints are prone to developing osteoarthritis in those joints. For example, osteoarthritis may affect the hips, ankles, and feet of ballet dancers, the knees of soccer players, the hips of farmers, the elbows of riveters, and the hands and wrists of pneumatic tool operators. The cause is thought to be repetitive, high-

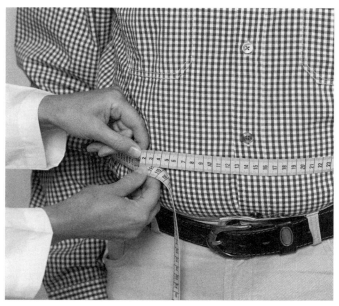

Being overweight can make your knees and hips susceptible to developing osteoarthritis. If you already have arthritis, losing weight can reduce pressure on your joints and help relieve your pain.

intensity stress leading to bone fatigue, microscopic fractures, and eventually cartilage breakdown.

By contrast, day-to-day use, even "overuse," of joints does not necessarily increase risk. For example, people who spend a lot of time using a keyboard are no more likely than others to develop osteoarthritis of the hands. And people with osteoarthritis in their hands do not necessarily have more of it in their dominant hand. If osteoarthritis were caused by overuse, it would logically occur more commonly in the hand you use most. So, simply using a joint frequently does not mean osteoarthritis is inevitable.

Even regular jogging on pavement does not predictably lead to osteoarthritis of the knee, perhaps because the large muscles in the legs tend to dampen the impact on joints. (In soccer, it's not the running, but more likely the twisting and torquing, that can injure cartilage in the knee and lead to osteoarthritis.) In fact, in some studies runners appear to have a lower rate of osteoarthritis than nonrunners—possibly because they are more likely to be fit and trim to start with.

Other diseases. Osteoarthritis can develop in a joint damaged by a related disease, such as rheumatoid arthritis, infectious arthritis, or gout (see "Other types of arthritis," page 44, and Table 1, page 46).

Osteoarthritis may also develop because of a growth abnormality. Such abnormalities include acromegaly (the irregular overgrowth of bone and cartilage because of abnormal production of growth hormone) and slipped capital femoral epiphysis (displacement of the growth plate at the top of the thighbone, where it joins the hip).

Osteoarthritis can also arise from certain hereditary metabolic diseases, such as hemochromatosis (the harmful accumulation of iron in tissues). Even hemophilia, in which blood does not clot properly, can lead to osteoarthritis as a result of repeated bleeding in the joint.

Symptoms of osteoarthritis

The symptoms of osteoarthritis usually develop over many years. Often, people first experience pain after engaging in strenuous activity or overusing a joint. The joint may be stiff in the morning, but after a few minutes of movement, it loosens up. Gradually, this stiffness becomes a routine part of waking up.

Cartilage is insensitive to pain, but the soft tissue around the joints is not. As more cartilage wears away, the soft tissue becomes increasingly irritated, even by slight movement. Some people have continual joint pain that interferes with sleep. Alternatively, the joint may be mildly tender, and movement may produce crepitus, a sensation of crackling or grating. In addition, gradual joint enlargement may interfere with normal mobility. Swelling may occur as synovial tissues become irritated or when inflammation develops. Pain is usually confined to the affected joint, although it may extend elsewhere.

Pain and stiffness in affected joints may slowly worsen over the years, but most people are able to lead normal lives.

Knee

Early in the process of knee osteoarthritis, the space between the tibia (shin bone) and the femur (thighbone) decreases as the cartilage wears away (see Figure 4, at left). Bone rubs on bone, and osteophytes can form. The result is pain, swelling, and stiffness. What starts out as discomfort after a period of disuse can progress to difficulty walking, climbing, bathing, and getting in and out of bed. There may be intermittent or steady pain, swelling or tenderness, and grinding or crunching sounds. For many people, the pain tends to worsen as muscles tire during the day.

Hip

The hip is a common site for osteoarthritis. Pain radiating to the buttocks or knees is often the most striking feature. You may also feel pain in the groin or radiating down the inside of the thigh or when you pivot or rotate the hip inward. Other symptoms of hip osteoarthritis include the following:

- stiffness after inactivity and first thing in the morning
- difficulty bending
- limping or other gait changes
- apparent shortness of the leg on the affected side
- difficulty with foot care
- groin pain when you get out of a chair
- difficulty getting in and out of a car.

Figure 4: Osteoarthritis of the knee

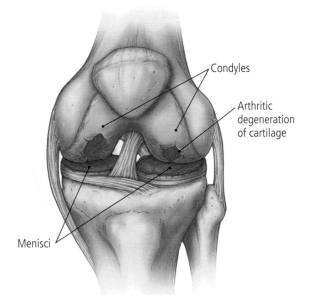

Condyles

Arthritic degeneration of cartilage

Menisci

Multiple factors contribute to the development of knee osteoarthritis. But once it begins, the wear and tear of repeated motion and weight placed on the joint may cause the cartilage there to degenerate more quickly than in some other joints. In this illustration, the articular cartilage of the condyles (knobs at the lower end of the thighbone) is degraded.

Spine

Osteoarthritis can affect the cervical spine (the neck) and the lumbar spine (lower back). The spine is a column of interlocking bones called vertebrae (see Figure 5, below). Each vertebra has a cylindrical body with a bony ring attached to its back surface. (The stack of rings forms the spinal canal, through which the spinal cord runs.) Spiky projections extend in several directions from the bony ring on each vertebra. Four of these connect with projections on vertebrae above and below at what are called facet joints. These joints give the spine stability and also allow it to bend. Facet joints can develop osteoarthritis. In the cervical spine, this may cause pain in your neck, shoulders, and arms. You may hear a crunching or grinding sound as you turn your head. In the lumbar spine, osteoarthritis can cause low back pain and limit motion. In both the cervical and lumbar spine, osteophytes can form. These may impinge on adjacent nerves and send pain radiating to your arms (if they are in the cervical spine) or down the buttocks or legs (if they are in the lumbar spine).

Hand

Certain joints of the hands (see Figure 6, page 10) are especially susceptible to osteoarthritis:

- The last joint before the nail (the distal interphalangeal, or DIP, joint) is the most common site for osteoarthritis of the hands. These joints sometimes develop osteophytes known as Heberden's nodes. Because the finger joints are close to the skin surface, osteophytes in this location tend to be more visible than when they occur in other joints. These bumps can be painful, red, and swollen, and they may interfere with your ability to bend and straighten your fingers. Over time, pain diminishes, but the bony protrusion remains.

Does knuckle cracking cause arthritis?

Cracking your knuckles may provoke an annoyed grimace from those around you, but it probably won't raise your risk for arthritis. That's the conclusion of several studies that compared rates of hand arthritis among habitual knuckle-crackers and people who didn't crack their knuckles.

The "pop" of a cracked knuckle is caused by bubbles bursting in the synovial fluid. The bubbles pop when you pull the bones apart, either by stretching the fingers or bending them backward, creating negative pressure.

- The joint at the base of the thumb, where it meets the wrist (the first carpometacarpal, or CMC, joint), is the second most common site of hand osteoarthritis.
- The middle joint of each finger (the proximal interphalangeal, or PIP, joints) can also develop osteoarthritis, causing the fingers to stiffen and swell. Osteophytes in these joints are called Bouchard's nodes.

Osteoarthritis of the hand often starts with stiffness and soreness of the affected joint, particularly in the morning. You may find that it's harder to pinch and that your joints crackle when you move them. As

Figure 5: A closer look at your lumbar vertebrae

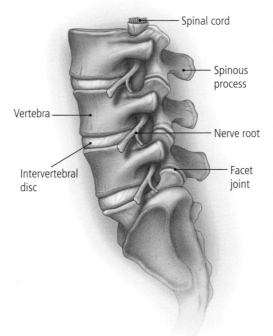

Spinal cord
Spinous process
Vertebra
Nerve root
Intervertebral disc
Facet joint

Each vertebra has a cylindrical body with a bony ring attached to it for the spinal cord to pass through. Each vertebra also has seven bony extensions, the largest of which is called the spinous process. Four smaller processes (called articular processes) connect with those of neighboring vertebrae at small joints known as facet joints. If you have osteoarthritis in your spine, it probably involves your facet joints.

Intervertebral discs, tucked between each pair of vertebrae, serve as shock absorbers. These can deteriorate with age, but that is a separate medical condition from osteoarthritis.

Figure 6: Inside the hand

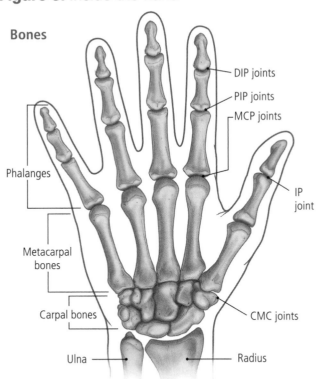

Bones

DIP joints
PIP joints
MCP joints
Phalanges
IP joint
Metacarpal bones
Carpal bones
CMC joints
Ulna
Radius

Under the skin, the hand's 27 bones and 34 muscles work in synchrony to perform a range of movements, from a powerful hammer blow to a gentle caress. Because the hand has so many bones, it also has many joints. Those most often affected by osteoarthritis are the distal interphalangeal (DIP) and proximal interphalangeal (PIP) joints in the fingers, and all the thumb's joints, including the first carpometacarpal (CMC) joint near the wrist.

the condition worsens, the pain at the base of your thumb may become more of a problem, and your ability to grip may decrease even further. The entire area may seem unstable. People with osteoarthritis of the hand may eventually find it impossible to open jars, turn a key, write, or type.

Many people with osteoarthritis of the hand find that, with age, their hands thicken and become stiff. Stiffness is gradually followed by pain or instability. In other people, the pain and stiffness of hand osteoarthritis may subside over time, despite marked bony enlargement typical of the disease.

Feet

As in the hand, certain joints of the foot are more susceptible than others. Joints in the midfoot and ankle may be affected, but the most common site is the joint where the big toe meets the rest of the foot (the first metatarsophalangeal, or MTP, joint).

Over time, osteoarthritic joints may stiffen and become sore, making walking difficult. Some people develop osteophytes at the joint.

In some people with osteoarthritis at the first MTP joint, the bones become misaligned, forcing the toe to bend toward the others. This contributes to the formation of a bunion—a lump on the side of the foot at the base of the big toe. Bunions can be painful and make it difficult to wear shoes. ♥

Diagnosing osteoarthritis

If you have joint pain, you may wonder what type of doctor you should see. It's best to start with your primary care physician, who can make an evaluation and, in most cases, manage your treatment. Your primary care doctor may refer you to one or more specialists, such as a rheumatologist, physiatrist, physical therapist, or orthopedic surgeon, depending on your condition and your needs (see "Specialists who treat osteoarthritis," below).

Diagnosing osteoarthritis can be challenging because numerous conditions can cause joint discomfort. When making a diagnosis, doctors rely heavily on your description of symptoms and other relevant information, plus a physical examination. That's why you should prepare for your appointment by making a list of your symptoms and the circumstances under which they occur. Do you notice them during or after a particular activity? Are your symptoms worse first thing in the morning?

Primary care doctors can usually determine at the first visit whether the problem is arthritis or some other musculoskeletal problem, such as bursitis, tendinitis, or a meniscal tear. But it may take several visits for your physician to make a more specific diagnosis regarding the particular type of arthritis (see "Other types of arthritis," page 44, and Table 1, page 46, for more information on those conditions). While this delay can be frustrating for you and your family, charting the course of your symptoms is often the only way a doctor can accurately diagnose arthritis.

When symptoms don't fit the usual pattern for primary osteoarthritis, further investigation may be necessary. For example, if the doctor suspects you have another type of arthritis, you may need a blood test or

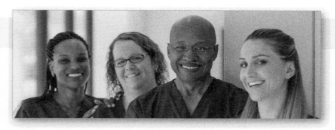

with osteoarthritis, orthopedic surgeons perform joint replacement and other types of surgeries. Most orthopedists specialize in certain joints, such as the knee, hip, shoulder, hand, ankle, or spine.

Physical therapists. These medical professionals focus on helping to restore or maintain your ability to move and walk. For people with osteoarthritis, they often oversee a program of exercises to strengthen muscles, build endurance, and improve balance. Physical therapy supplements but does not replace care by a medical doctor.

Occupational therapists. These medical professionals help to improve your ability to perform activities of daily living, such as dressing, bathing, and eating. They tend to focus on physical function, especially involving the hand and wrist. Like physical therapy, occupational therapy is given in addition to medical care.

Specialists who treat osteoarthritis

Most of the time, a primary care doctor can manage osteoarthritis with standard treatments. However, if symptoms don't improve or if they get worse—or if the doctor suspects some other cause of joint problems besides osteoarthritis—you may receive a referral to a specialist.

Rheumatologists. These doctors specialize in diagnosing and treating diseases of the musculoskeletal system—that is, the body's joints, muscles, and bones—and systemic autoimmune diseases. Diseases they treat include osteoarthritis, rheumatoid arthritis, gout, tendinitis, and lupus.

Physiatrists (also called rehabilitation physicians). These doctors treat injuries or illnesses that affect how you move, including osteoarthritis. A physiatrist will make an assessment and put together an individualized treatment program, which will most likely include other members of the health care team, such as physical and occupational therapists.

Orthopedic surgeons (also called orthopedists). These doctors focus on injuries and diseases of the musculoskeletal system. They are trained in all aspects of diagnosis and treatment, with an emphasis on surgery. For people other diagnostic tests. X-rays can be used to establish a diagnosis of osteoarthritis, although early arthritic changes may not be pronounced enough to show up on the image. This means that you can have a normal-looking x-ray and still have osteoarthritis.

Your medical history

Your symptoms—what they are, when they first began, and how they've changed over time—provide important clues to whether the problem is osteoarthritis or another type of arthritis, such as rheumatoid arthritis. Your doctor will need to know about the following:

- the type of joint symptoms (such as pain or stiffness)
- the effect of activity (such as increased pain or relief of stiffness during or after a particular activity)
- the general pattern of joint symptoms (whether they started gradually or suddenly, worsened over time or stayed about the same, migrated from one joint to another, or fluctuated in intensity)
- any other symptoms (such as fever, fatigue, weight loss, skin problems, or bowel problems)
- events that occurred near the time the symptoms first appeared (such as viral illness, bacterial infection, injury, vaccination, new medication, or change in activity)
- the time of day that joint symptoms are worst (for instance, brief morning stiffness and night pain are typical of osteoarthritis)
- the presence or absence of joint swelling, redness, or warmth
- previous episodes of similar symptoms
- any family history of arthritis or rheumatic disease.

Pain and stiffness

Pain is a subjective experience that's often difficult for people to describe, quantify, or even pinpoint. Chronic arthritis produces aching pain when the affected joints are moved, as opposed to the burning or prickling pain unrelated to motion that typifies nerve disorders such as diabetic neuropathy. Most people can describe the location of pain in small joints, such as the hands or feet. However, with large joints, the pain is generally

When to see a doctor without delay

Because arthritis is rarely a medical emergency, you can usually schedule a routine appointment for evaluation. However, certain situations and symptoms demand immediate attention. These include the following:

- joint injury, especially if the joint cannot function or there is a feeling of instability; this may require orthopedic surgery
- joint pain accompanied by broader systemic problems such as fever, rash, fatigue, headache, or weight loss; this can indicate other autoimmune diseases, chronic infection, or cancer
- sudden severe pain in one or a few joints; this can indicate joint infection or gout
- neurologic symptoms, such as numbness or pain in the hands or legs, radiating from the neck, or in the lower back; this may indicate nerve compression.

more diffuse and may radiate, making it difficult to say where it originates. For example, hip arthritis may cause pain in the groin, thighs, buttocks, or even knees.

People often describe vague muscle aches as stiffness, but rheumatologists use the term more specifically for joint discomfort when a person attempts to move. Stiffness is the tendency of a joint not to move easily and may be prominent even when joint pain is not.

The duration of stiffness in the morning or after any period of inactivity can help doctors distinguish osteoarthritis from rheumatoid arthritis and other types of arthritis. Mild morning stiffness is common in osteoarthritis and resolves after a few minutes of activity. In rheumatoid arthritis, however, morning stiffness may not begin to improve for an hour or longer. Occasionally, morning stiffness is the first symptom of rheumatoid arthritis. Sometimes people with osteoarthritis notice more stiffness during the day after resting for an hour or so.

To understand the intensity of your pain, your doctor may ask you to rate it according to a pain scale (see Figure 7, page 13). In addition, he or she will want to know about the nature and duration of your symptoms. Pain and stiffness that develop gradually and intermittently over several months or years suggest osteoarthritis. By contrast, rheumatoid arthritis or another inflammatory arthritis may cause pain, stiffness, and fatigue that worsen in as little as several weeks or a few months. Sudden pain over a day or two is more likely a result of injury or fracture, and pain that intensifies over several hours is typical of bacterial infection or gout.

Physical examination

Because many other disorders can masquerade as arthritis, a complete physical examination is a necessary part of the diagnostic process. During your visit, the doctor watches how you move and gains information from a visual assessment of how you use your joints. He or she may ask you to take a few steps, move your hands and arms, and so forth. The doctor will also move your joints through their range of motion to detect any pain, resistance, unusual sounds, or instability, and will examine your joints for abnormalities.

Swelling. An inflamed synovial membrane often produces mild joint swelling. People may describe a sensation of tightness or fullness inside the joint, or it may feel tender. Doctors describe the joint as feeling "boggy" or soft to the touch. Marked swelling usually indicates excessive joint fluid, a sign of inflammation or perhaps bleeding into the joint.

Enlargement. Enlargement of a joint is not the same as swelling. Bony enlargement without joint swelling feels hard to the touch and is not usually tender. This is a classic sign of osteoarthritis.

Limited motion. Doctors assess joint mobility in two ways: active range of motion in which the person voluntarily moves the joints, and passive range of motion in which the examiner moves the person's joints. By comparing active and passive movement, doctors can often determine whether the cause is muscle weakness, bursitis, or tendinitis (in which case the joint has wider range of motion during passive movement), or whether the problem is with the joint itself. Doctors listen and feel for crepitus, a crunching or grating sensation and sound caused by rough surfaces rubbing together inside the joint.

Limited spine flexibility. This may indicate osteoarthritis or another type of arthritis, such as ankylosing spondylitis. To evaluate spine flexibility, the doctor may ask you to stand and bend forward and backward, lean from side to side, and twist your torso.

Diagnostic tests

In addition to a medical history and physical examination, your physician may need an x-ray of the affected joint to help make a diagnosis of osteoarthritis. Blood tests, imaging, and a procedure called arthrocentesis may also be recommended to rule out other types of the disease, such as rheumatoid arthritis (see "Diagnosing rheumatoid arthritis," page 45).

Blood tests

Although these tests are not used to diagnose osteoarthritis, doctors may use them to rule out other forms of arthritis.

Figure 7: How much does it hurt? Keeping track

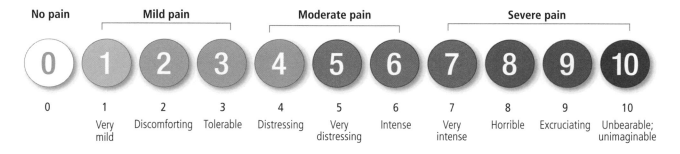

A pain record is useful. For two weeks before your doctor's appointment, keep a record of the intensity of your pain on a scale of 1 to 10, its duration, its characteristics, and anything that makes it worse or better. Your doctor will use this information in diagnosis.

Antibody tests. When rheumatoid arthritis is a possibility, many doctors order tests for rheumatoid factor (RF) and anti-cyclic citrullinated peptide (anti-CCP). An antinuclear antibody test may be used if lupus or related conditions are under consideration.

Erythrocyte sedimentation rate and C-reactive protein. These blood tests are general measurements for inflammation of any kind: the higher the result, the more severe the inflammation. Most people with osteoarthritis have normal values, but those who have inflammatory conditions, such as rheumatoid arthritis, usually have elevated levels.

Serum uric acid test. This test measures the level of uric acid in the blood, which is usually elevated in people with gout.

Other blood tests. A person's history may indicate the need to test for Lyme disease or other infections, which can cause reactive arthritis and other types of infectious arthritis.

Imaging tests

Doctors may order one or more imaging tests to better evaluate your joints. The type of test ordered depends on the suspected diagnosis.

X-rays. Most forms of arthritis can cause joint abnormalities that are visible on x-rays (see Figure 8, at right), including a reduction in the joint space and increased bone density (sclerosis). Bone cysts near the joint, another sign of osteoarthritis, may also be visible. But in most cases, such changes can't be detected until months or even years after symptoms begin. Sometimes the changes are reasonably specific and suggest a particular kind of arthritis. In other cases, they are more general. For example, bone damage (erosion) is often found in rheumatoid arthritis and may occur in gout, but the damage from each of these differs enough in appearance that a radiologist can usually tell them apart.

Often, the changes revealed in x-rays bear little relationship to the actual symptoms, especially in osteoarthritis. An x-ray showing large osteophytes on the finger joints may belong to a woman with nothing more than occasional mild aching in her hands, while an x-ray revealing much less dramatic abnormalities may be that of a woman who can no longer work in the garden because of hand pain.

Further complicating matters, osteoarthritis and rheumatoid arthritis may appear quite similar on x-ray examination in their later stages. In rheumatoid arthritis, the inflamed tissue (pannus) erodes cartilage, and in many cases, the joint damage eventually leads to secondary osteoarthritis, even after the inflammation subsides.

Magnetic resonance imaging (MRI). In evaluating people with joint problems, this test can help doctors assess soft tissues, cartilage, tendons, and joint inflammation. It's also quite good for detecting spinal cord and nerve root compression that can be caused by degenerative disc disease in the spine. In addition, MRI has been used to help diagnose rheumatoid arthritis.

Ultrasound. This technique uses sound waves to assess fluid in soft tissues and abnormalities in muscles or tendons. Many doctors are using ultrasound to identify inflammation and joint damage and to guide procedures such as arthrocentesis. Researchers are studying whether ultrasound can also detect erosions in rheumatoid arthritis and other types of arthritis.

Computed tomography (CT). CT imaging uses

Figure 8: Osteoarthritis of the hip

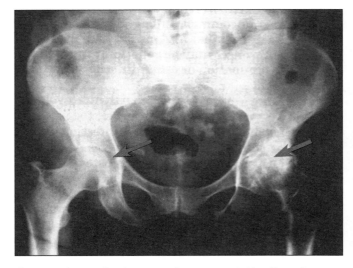

This x-ray shows what happens when osteoarthritis affects the hip—in this case, the patient's left hip (shown on the right side of the image). Compared with the visible outline of the ball-and-socket joint on the opposite side, the joint on this side has noticeably deteriorated.

a rotating x-ray tube housed in a doughnut-shaped machine to show thin x-ray slices of your anatomy. A computer then assembles these slices into a three-dimensional picture. Doctors occasionally order CT scans to detect hidden fractures, bone infection, or other abnormalities of bone.

Arthrocentesis

In this diagnostic procedure, which is most commonly performed when a person develops sudden or unexplained joint swelling, a physician uses a needle to remove some of the synovial fluid for examination. Excess synovial fluid may indicate a bacterial infection in the joint, crystal deposits, injury, bleeding into the joint, or synovial inflammation. In cases where arthritis symptoms are relatively mild, arthrocentesis may help the doctor determine whether you have osteoarthritis (which tends to have minimal or only mild inflammation) or inflammatory joint disease (such as rheumatoid arthritis or gout).

Physicians can often get a good idea of whether the problem is inflammatory by the appearance of the fluid. Normally, it's translucent and pale-to-medium yellow. Significant inflammation may produce a deep yellow or greenish-yellow opaque fluid. Cloudy fluid may be a sign of crystals or infection.

A laboratory technician or physician examines the fluid under a microscope for crystals that indicate gout or similar disorders. Your doctor may request other laboratory tests on the fluid, such as a white blood cell count; a large number of white blood cells could indicate either infection or severe inflammation.

Aside from its diagnostic role, arthrocentesis itself is often beneficial because removing some of the excess synovial fluid can relieve pain and pressure. In addition, medications, such as corticosteroids, can be injected into the joint after fluid is removed (see "Corticosteroid injections," page 23). ♦

Treating osteoarthritis without surgery

Damaged cartilage does not heal, and there is currently no cure for osteoarthritis. But treatment can greatly improve your quality of life by relieving pain, protecting your joints, and increasing your range of motion. Therapy usually involves a combination of strategies, including physical and occupational therapy, ongoing exercise, assistive devices, weight loss (if you are overweight), pain medications, and joint injections. There are also complementary strategies that some people find helpful. In some cases, more aggressive treatment with surgery may be needed (see "Surgical treatment of osteoarthritis," page 35).

Physical and occupational therapy

Physical therapy and occupational therapy are the cornerstones of treatment for osteoarthritis. Even though they cannot restore damaged cartilage, they can help you strengthen the muscles supporting your joints, increase flexibility and range of motion in those joints, and help protect them from further damage. Physical therapists and occupational therapists can help in all of these areas.

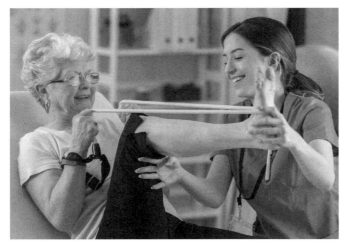

Physical therapists often work with people who have arthritis. Among other things, they work on helping you to strengthen the muscles that support arthritic joints.

Both physical and occupational therapists will start by thoroughly evaluating your pain, functional ability, strength, and endurance levels. They will then focus on restoring or maintaining physical function by designing an individualized treatment program for you. But there are differences between these approaches.

Physical therapy helps people to reduce pain and restore and maintain mobility, usually with an exercise program. For a person with osteoarthritis, a physical therapist will design a specially tailored exercise program that builds muscle to support affected joints and helps restore and maintain flexibility. The therapist may also use manual therapy techniques, including stretching and myofascial release (the application of gentle pressure to soft tissues to improve flexibility and mobility in an area). Physical therapists may educate you about optimal posture and body mechanics and suggest assistive devices to help protect your joints.

Physical therapy sessions typically last 30 to 60 minutes and can take place at a hospital or outpatient clinic, in the therapist's office, or in your home. Some activities can be done on your own; others require the therapist's assistance. (For exercises to preserve mobility and increase strength, see "Exercise," page 27.)

To get the most out of physical therapy and maintain the gains you made while working one-on-one with the therapist, you must continue doing exercises at home on a regular basis indefinitely.

Occupational therapy focuses on helping people perform day-to-day tasks and activities at home (such as preparing meals, maintaining personal hygiene, and using utensils) and at work (such as typing). Occupational therapists often work with people who have arthritis in the hands or wrists. For a person with osteoarthritis, an occupational therapist may offer suggestions about how to better perform and manage everyday tasks. He or she will also give you advice about ways to ease pressure on your joints and may provide you with special assistive devices, such as a splint, brace, sling, elastic bandage, or cane, to reduce pressure on tender joints and protect them from further injury. (Strategies to protect joints and helpful gadgets are described in the Special Section, "Self-care strategies for coping with arthritis," page 26.)

Assistive devices

Splints or braces for joints affected by osteoarthritis may relieve some symptoms. Because it is important to get the right brace or splint and the correct fit, be sure to consult a doctor, physical therapist, or occupational therapist before buying any kind of assistive device. Even if you use a splint or brace, it is important to take steps to protect your joints (see "Joint protection strategies," page 31). Adaptive aids may also be useful (see "Helpful gadgets," page 32).

Knees

If you have early, mild knee arthritis with sudden

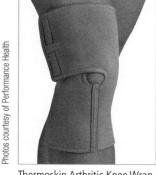

Thermoskin Arthritic Knee Wrap

flare-ups, a simple knee wrap made of neoprene or elastic (see photo, at left, for an example) may help to relieve pain. Because the wrap itself doesn't provide much support, any benefit is thought to be due to improvements in the knee's movement and position.

If you have knee osteoarthritis affecting only one side of the joint, a different type of brace known as an unloader brace (see photo, above right, for an example) may help by taking some of the pressure off that part of the knee and redistributing the weight (or load) to other parts. These braces change the angle of the knee joint using special hinges to reduce force on the joint. However, many people find this type of brace cumbersome or uncomfortable.

Another kind of brace is used in people with arthritis affecting the joint underneath the kneecap. Consisting of a sleeve with a cutout at the kneecap and pads below and to the outside, this brace is designed

to reduce compression of the kneecap, improve its alignment, and prevent side-to-side shifting.

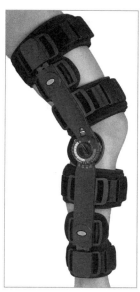

Rolyan Defender Post-Op Knee Brace

Foot orthotics, or specialized shoe inserts, may also prove helpful for people with knee arthritis because flat feet or other foot problems can affect the alignment of the ankle and knee, placing additional stress on the joints. Shock-absorbing insoles made of a gel-like material may also help reduce the symptoms of knee osteoarthritis. One study showed that these shoe inserts reduced the force of each step by 42% and improved symptoms in 78% of the people who used them. You can purchase ready-made orthotics from companies such as Powerstep, Superfeet, and Spenco. If those don't work, a podiatrist or physical therapist can order custom-made foot orthotics.

Everyday footwear also makes a difference. Shoes should be supportive and have good shock absorption, cushioning, and arch support, as well as adequate room in the toe box. Going barefoot, even around the house, may be uncomfortable for people with knee arthritis, so wear supportive shoes, sandals, or slippers. If you don't want to wear street shoes in the house, use a pair of home-only shoes.

Another option for taking pressure off arthritic knees is to use a cane (see "Easing the strain with a cane," page 18).

Ankles

If you have ankle osteoarthritis, you may change the way you walk to compensate for pain and limited movement, which can put stress on your other joints. Ankle supports are designed to improve balance and normalize your

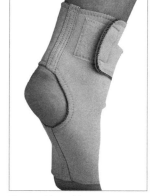

Thermoskin Ankle Wrap

walking patterns. Devices range from an ankle brace (see photo, page 17), to a semirigid foot orthotic, to shoe modifications (such as a lateral wedge insert or rocker sole and cushioned heel), to custom-made, molded-plastic orthotics for people with more severe disease. Ask your doctor or therapist which is right for you. If your arthritis is severe, he or she may order one of various forms of immobilization boots, which can be effective when used for walking and standing.

Feet

If you have arthritis in your feet, a podiatrist or physical therapist may be able to provide orthotics, recommend special shoes, or suggest other treatments to reduce pain and improve your ability to function.

Hips

Except in rare situations, using a brace to support the hip doesn't seem to be helpful. A straight cane, on the other hand, can help quite a bit. When you stand without leaning on a cane, the pressure on the hip increases as much as four times. If you have pain in both hips, you should use the cane on the side opposite to the hip that is the most troublesome, and alternate sides as needed (see "Easing the strain with a cane," below).

Hands

Hand splints can provide pain relief, improve function, or realign the joints of the hand to a more anatomically correct position. They come in a wide range of materials and forms. A prefabricated splint from the drugstore or medical supply store works well for certain hand problems. Other conditions require custom-made splints, which are usually made of plastic material that can be heated and then molded to fit around the contours of the hand. Whether you use a prefabricated or custom-made splint, a medical professional—such as a doctor, nurse, or occupational therapist who specializes in hands—can help you choose the most appropriate splint and adjust it correctly.

Easing the strain with a cane

For something so low-tech and simple in design, a cane performs complex functions. You hold the cane in the hand opposite the side that needs support, about four inches to the side of your stronger leg. This redistributes weight to improve stability, helps reduce demand on muscles that may be weak, and takes the load off weight-bearing structures such as the hip, knee, and spine.

A cane can help you maintain mobility and ward off further disability if you have arthritis of the knee or hip, as well as assist in recovery after surgery. So don't let self-consciousness stop you from using a cane if your doctor recommends that you try one.

A physical therapist or other clinician can help you select a cane, check that it's the proper height, and show you how to use it. He or she may also suggest certain muscle-strengthening exercises before you start walking with your cane.

Canes are available at medical supply stores and pharmacies, through specialty catalogs, and on the Internet. They generally

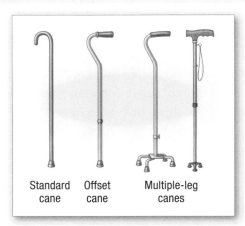

Standard cane   Offset cane   Multiple-leg canes

come in standard, offset, and multiple-legged versions. Government or private insurance usually covers the cost of a basic cane if you have a written prescription from your doctor.

Standard canes. These are low-tech, lightweight, and generally inexpensive. They usually come with a curved or T-shaped handle and a rubber-capped tip at the bottom. Many people find that a T-shaped handle is more comfortable than a curved one. A standard model is good for people who need help with balance but don't need the cane to bear a lot of weight.

Offset canes. The upper shaft of an offset cane bends outward, and the handle grip is usually flat—often a good choice for people whose hands are weak or who need a cane that bears more weight than the standard type.

Multi-leg canes. Multiple legs offer considerable support and allow the cane to stand on its own when not in use. One drawback to using such a cane is that for maximum support, you must plant all the legs solidly on the ground. Doing so takes time and can slow the pace of walking.

Static splints hold the joint in one position, while dynamic splints allow movement. Some are designed to help lengthen tightened joint capsules, muscles, and tendons. Others, which feature elastic or spring-loaded parts, make up for missing motion in the hands and wrists caused by muscle weakness or nerve damage.

Several types of splints are designed to address problems with the finger joints. These include a figure-eight splint and a prefabricated "oval-eight" splint, which allow you to fully bend the finger joint closest to the hand but protect the joint from hyperextension. In addition, custom-made splints prevent the joint from bending backward and from moving sideways. A "gutter" splint may be fabricated to immobilize only the joints that are painful or swollen. Various custom-made splints can also be made to help with problems at the base of the thumb. Your doctor or therapist will help you determine which one is most appropriate.

Wrists

There are several options for wrist splinting, depending on your needs. For people with early disease, simple off-the-shelf elastic or neoprene splints may be enough to reduce pain and improve function. If your arthritis is more severe, custom-molded splints may be a better option because they provide more joint control. The type of splint and materials used in its fabrication will depend on the demands of the wrist. For example, a laborer will need sturdier material than someone who works at a desk.

Spine

Braces aren't used for arthritis in the spine. But in some cases, a traction device may be helpful. Osteoarthritis in the spine can lead to compression of nerves, which can cause pain that shoots down the arm (in the case of cervical spine arthritis) or the legs (with lumbar spine arthritis). Traction devices come in various configurations. For example, a physical therapist might position you in a chair with a strap around your head. The device pulls your head up slightly and holds you in that stretched position for 15 to 20 minutes. This lengthens the spine to increase the space between joints, which can provide temporary relief. The units

are also available for home use, but should be tried only after you've received detailed instructions how to use them.

If neck pain is severe or if you have difficulty holding your head up because of weakened muscles, your doctor or physical therapist might recommend a neck collar. This can also help if you have pain at night when turning your head. However, you should not wear a neck collar all day, or your neck muscles will weaken even more. During the day, you should wear the collar only for an hour or two at a time.

Drug treatment

Although no drug will cure or reverse the progression of osteoarthritis, there are some that can alleviate pain and inflammation. Medications are best used as part of a comprehensive treatment plan that includes other pain relief strategies, such as physical therapy, exercise, use of assistive devices, protecting your joints from injury or overuse, and other measures that are described in the Special Section, "Self-care strategies for coping with arthritis," page 26. (An overview of drugs for osteoarthritis appears in the Appendix.)

Topical pain relievers

Topical pain relievers, which are applied to the skin, offer one option for mild pain relief. You can use these alone or in combination with oral pain relievers. They come in a variety of forms, including creams, gels, ointments, and patches. Some require a prescription, while others are available over the counter.

Over-the-counter topicals. There are three types of topical pain reliever that can be bought without a prescription—capsaicin, salicylates, and counterirritants.

- *Capsaicin* is the substance in chili peppers that makes them spicy. Ironically, this substance also has pain-relieving qualities when applied to the skin. It works by blocking the release of a chemical messenger called substance P, which transmits pain sensations to the brain. Capsaicin comes in a cream (Capzasin, Zostrix) to rub on the skin. It causes a slight burning sensation and may require a week or two of regular use to produce any noticeable effects. If you try it, avoid touching any mucous membrane around your mouth, nose, or eyes after applying the cream, in order to avoid irritating sensitive tissues.

- *Salicylates,* such as Aspercreme, Bengay, Flexall, and Salonpas, contain a chemical similar to the one in aspirin that blocks the release of prostaglandins (substances that promote inflammation). These creams may provide temporary pain relief. People who are sensitive to aspirin should talk to their doctor before using these products.
- *Counterirritants* create a temporary heating or cooling sensation, which may interfere with the transmission of pain signals and distract you from pain. They contain ingredients such as menthol, eucalyptus, camphor oil, or wintergreen. Common ones are Biofreeze and Icy Hot.

Prescription topicals. Some prescription drugs also come in topical forms, including diclofenac and lidocaine.

- *Diclofenac* is a nonsteroidal anti-inflammatory drug (see "NSAIDs," page 21). It is available in a gel (Voltaren), patch (Flector Patch), and drops or spray (Pennsaid). People who can't tolerate oral NSAIDs because of the stomach irritation these drugs cause may be able to use one of the topical versions instead. Because it is delivered through the skin, there is a lower chance for gastrointestinal and other side effects. However, some of the medicine is absorbed into the body, so the potential for side effects is not completely eliminated.
- *Lidocaine* is an anesthetic. It stops nerves from sending pain signals, creating a numbing sensation. A lidocaine patch may be used to relieve arthritis pain. However, insurance will not cover the cost of a lidocaine patch for osteoarthritis.

While the notion of applying medicine right to the

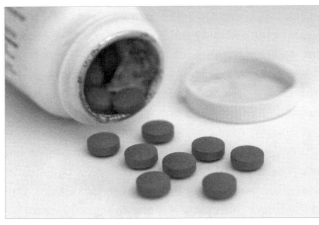

Over-the-counter pain relievers such as aspirin, ibuprofen, and naproxen can reduce arthritis pain and low-level inflammation. Acetaminophen is less effective for osteoarthritis.

spot that hurts has intuitive appeal, there are some doubts about how well such remedies work. With something as subjective as pain, it can be hard for researchers to figure out just how effective a treatment is. For example, an ointment that provides a soothing sensation might be considered effective in some studies, even if the relief isn't substantial enough to change an individual's overall perception of pain as measured on a pain scale. And the placebo effect—the benefit that comes from a person's expectations rather than the treatment itself—is a major complicating factor. On the other hand, there's no question that active medicine can penetrate the skin and get into the body; how much is absorbed is a separate question.

Acetaminophen

To relieve the pain and stiffness of osteoarthritis, the first step is usually an over-the-counter pill. Doctors often recommend acetaminophen (Tylenol) first because it relieves mild pain for some people and is easy on the stomach. However, the results of several studies call into question just how effective it really is for osteoarthritis. One study reviewed 12 trials that compared acetaminophen to a placebo for spinal pain or osteoarthritis of the hip or knee. The researchers found that acetaminophen was not effective for low back pain and provided only minimal short-term pain relief for people with osteoarthritis in the hip or knee.

Results of at least one study suggested that acetaminophen may be more effective when combined with ibuprofen (Advil or Motrin). The study, published in the journal *Annals of the Rheumatic Diseases,* found that people with knee osteoarthritis who took a combination pill for slightly over three months had better pain relief than those taking acetaminophen alone.

Acetaminophen, like any drug, has its own risks—

especially for the liver. According to the American Association for the Study of Liver Diseases, each year about 50,000 emergency room visits and 500 fatalities are attributed to acetaminophen overdose—at least half of which are unintentional. Considering that millions of people take acetaminophen for pain relief every day, the number of people with acetaminophen-related liver failure is relatively small. Still, it remains the most common form of acute liver failure in the United States.

To avoid an accidental poisoning, don't exceed the recommended maximum, which is generally set at 3 grams (3,000 milligrams) per day—the equivalent of six extra-strength Tylenol tablets. According to the FDA, liver damage may occur if you regularly take more than 4 grams (4,000 milligrams) a day or if you drink three or more alcoholic beverages a day while taking acetaminophen. Remember that acetaminophen is often included in other drugs, such as cough and cold medications, so it's important to read the labels carefully.

NSAIDs

Nonsteroidal anti-inflammatory drugs (NSAIDs) are generally considered more effective than acetaminophen in treating osteoarthritis because they not only relieve pain, but also reduce inflammation that contributes to pain, swelling, and stiffness.

The arsenal of NSAIDs has grown over the years to include about 20 different drugs. Among them are such well-known medications as aspirin, ibuprofen (including Advil and Motrin), and naproxen (including Aleve and Naprosyn). They are available in both prescription and nonprescription strengths. These drugs reduce pain and inflammation by blocking the production of prostaglandins, leukotrienes, and other chemicals. For many people with arthritis, they are more effective than acetaminophen, especially during flare-ups of symptoms. As noted earlier, some research has shown that a combination of acetaminophen and ibuprofen may bring more relief than acetaminophen alone.

The most common side effects of NSAIDs are stomach problems, including gastrointestinal bleeding and ulcers, often occurring without warning. That's because NSAIDs not only block the COX-2 enzyme (which causes pain and inflammation), but also inhibit the helpful COX-1 enzyme (which helps protect the stomach lining from the corrosive effects of stomach acids and digestive enzymes). It's estimated that NSAIDs contribute to as many as 16,500 deaths and 100,000 hospitalizations in the United States each year.

Most of the time, gastrointestinal complications can be avoided—but you and your doctor must work together to determine your risk of experiencing them. The older you are, the higher your chances of developing bleeding and ulcers. You're also at higher risk if you have had ulcers in the past, have rheumatoid arthritis, or are taking a blood thinner or corticosteroids. Prolonged use and higher doses of NSAIDs also increase the risk. And some NSAIDs are more likely than others to cause ulcers; for example, aspirin (including Anacin and Bayer) and indomethacin (Indocin) appear to have the highest risk. If you are in a high-risk group, avoid NSAIDs if possible, and try other pain relief strategies.

If taking NSAIDs produces stomach upset but not a bleeding ulcer, good initial strategies are to reduce the dose of the NSAID you're taking, try an entirely different pain reliever (such as acetaminophen), or switch to a drug such as celecoxib (Cele-

▶ ## More potent painkillers

Occasionally, arthritis pain requires a stronger painkiller, such as tramadol (Ultram) or a combination of acetaminophen with codeine (Tylenol No. 3), an opiate medication. Usually, people take these medications intermittently for short periods (a week or so at a time). But if other therapies are not effective or are not tolerated, these prescription painkillers can be taken on a long-term basis. However, side effects may limit their use, and opiate addiction is a major concern. Tramadol commonly causes sleepiness and gastrointestinal symptoms, while codeine may cause constipation, nausea, and sleepiness. When opioid medications are used, they will be started at the lowest possible dose that is effective. The CDC recommends that doctors evaluate the benefits and harms within one to four weeks of starting opioid therapy for chronic pain. After that, an evaluation should be made at least every three months to make sure the benefits outweigh any harms.

brex; see "COX-2 inhibitors," below), which is more selective for COX-2 and therefore might be better tolerated. Nabumetone (Relafen), although not officially a COX-2 selective agent, is relatively selective for COX-2 and would be a better choice than a traditional NSAID such as indomethacin if stomach upset is a problem. Other more selective NSAIDs to consider, as they may be more easily tolerated, are meloxicam (Mobic) and diclofenac (Cataflam, Voltaren, Zorvolex).

If these strategies don't work, talk with your doctor about combining your NSAID with a drug that reduces stomach acid. These include histamine blockers such as cimetidine (Tagamet) and ranitidine (Zantac), as well as proton-pump inhibitors such as esomeprazole (Nexium), lansoprazole (Prevacid), and omeprazole (Prilosec). Some combination drugs (such as Arthrotec, Prevacid NapraPAC, and Vimovo) provide both an NSAID and an acid-reducing medication.

You should be aware that NSAIDs can increase your risk for a heart attack or stroke (see "NSAIDs and the risk for heart attacks and strokes," at right). If you have gastrointestinal, kidney, or heart problems, talk to your doctor before taking NSAIDs.

Whether you have risk factors or not, to be on the safe side, do not use NSAIDs on a daily basis except under the supervision of a doctor. Also take time at each doctor's visit to reassess the medication you are using for your arthritis. All too often, people take more medication than they really need. Other pain relief strategies might be used in combination with the drugs so you can lower the dose.

COX-2 inhibitors

COX-2 inhibitors were designed to be more selective in their effects than traditional NSAIDs. As their name implies, these drugs inhibit only the COX-2 enzyme involved in pain and inflammation, while sparing the COX-1 enzyme that protects the stomach lining. As such, they are able to relieve pain as well as the strongest NSAIDs, while causing less stomach irritation (although the risk of this side effect isn't eliminated). However, two of these drugs were later found to significantly increase the risk of heart attack

and stroke, which led the FDA to remove them from the market. The remaining one, celecoxib (Celebrex), poses the same (lower) risk for heart attack and stroke as the traditional NSAIDs ibuprofen and naproxen.

Atypical pain medications

Some drugs that are not typical pain medications may also provide relief. For example, the drug gabapentin (Neurontin) is an antiseizure drug for people with epilepsy. It can also be used to treat nerve pain, and it is approved by the FDA for the type of nerve pain that can occur in some people after having shingles. Doctors also prescribe it for other chronic pain conditions, such as osteoarthritis, although these uses are considered off-label, meaning they aren't specifically approved by the FDA for these conditions.

Another drug that may be used for osteoarthritis is the antidepressant duloxetine (Cymbalta). This drug is FDA-approved to treat chronic musculoskeletal pain, which may include osteoarthritis.

NSAIDs and the risk for heart attacks and strokes

In 2005, the FDA warned that taking NSAIDs can increase risk for heart attack and stroke. In 2015, the agency strengthened the warning on all NSAIDs except aspirin. The concern about this risk first came to light with the COX-2 inhibitor rofecoxib (Vioxx), which was taken off the market in 2004. While other NSAIDs remain available, they carry the FDA warning, which notes that

• serious side effects can occur even within a few weeks of starting regular use of an NSAID

• the risk may increase with long-term use of an NSAID

• people who have heart disease are at greatest risk.

If you have heart disease or are at risk for it, talk to your doctor about the safest NSAID to take or whether you should avoid these drugs altogether. (Note: Low-dose aspirin, which helps prevent clotting, is still recommended for some people who have had a heart attack. People who regularly take aspirin to prevent a heart attack or stroke and also take another NSAID for pain relief should take the aspirin first, then wait 30 to 60 minutes before taking the additional drug. Otherwise, the blood-thinning effect of the aspirin is diminished.)

Corticosteroid injections

If your joints feel warm and swollen (a sign of inflammation), your doctor may remove a small amount of joint fluid and then inject a combination of a corticosteroid and an anesthetic, such as lidocaine. The pain-relieving effect of the anesthetic kicks in right away, while the corticosteroid takes a bit longer to start working. This procedure can relieve inflammation quickly, and the effects may last from several weeks to several months. This approach is used almost exclusively for severe symptoms associated with signs of inflammation, especially for osteoarthritis of the knee. Doctors limit corticosteroid injections to no more than three or four per year—and only when absolutely necessary—because more frequent injections of these drugs can damage the joints and may increase the risk of infection.

Hyaluronate injections

Another therapy for osteoarthritis involves injecting a synthetic version of a substance that naturally lubricates joints—a treatment known as viscosupplementation. Just like the Tin Man in *The Wizard of Oz* needed a squirt of oil to loosen up his joints, shots of hyaluronic acid are meant to restore pain-free movement.

Hyaluronic acid is a natural component of synovial fluid. Over time, hyaluronic acid can break down, leading to pain and stiffness. Synthetic forms of hyaluronic acid (Hyalgan, Synvisc) can be injected directly into an osteoarthritic joint, theoretically restoring the lubricating qualities of synovial fluid.

This treatment is approved by the FDA for knee osteoarthritis. But the jury is still out on how effective it is. Several studies have examined viscosupplementation. Some of them have shown a small benefit, while others have found no difference when compared with placebo.

Possible side effects of viscosupplementation include pain at the injection site and infection.

Complementary therapies

Compared with conventional treatments, there is much less guidance on the usefulness of complementary therapies. Although hundreds of such therapies exist, only a few have actually proved to be effective when evaluated in rigorous studies.

So what should you do? Don't buy into any treatment that promises a cure. And be sure to ask questions: Do the claims rely only on testimonials from people who have tried the treatment, rather than on scientific studies? Are the promises extravagant? Do proponents advise not telling your doctor about the treatment? Do they suggest stopping medical treatment? Are the ingredients unidentified or "secret"? Is the source of your information selling the treatment? If your answer to any of these questions is "yes," your best response to the therapy may be "no."

The following are therapies with at least some evidence behind them. But before trying any complementary therapy, discuss it with your doctor to make sure it will support, rather than hinder, your arthritis management plan.

Glucosamine and chondroitin

Glucosamine and chondroitin are over-the-counter dietary supplements that may relieve pain in people with moderate to severe pain from osteoarthritis. Both are chemical components of cartilage, and in theory, supplements containing synthetic versions of these substances might help stop joint destruction and ease arthritis pain.

Over the years, some people with osteoarthritis have claimed to have less pain and stiffness when regularly taking these products. Some people swear by them. And some research suggests that such products may be helpful. A review of 43 studies that included a total of over 9,000 people who took either chondroitin (sometimes combined with glucosamine) or a placebo found that the supplement provided a small to moderate improvement in pain in the short term. The review was published in the *Cochrane Database of Systematic Reviews*.

If you're wondering whether you should take glucosamine and chondroitin, the answer is "it depends." If you are experiencing moderate to severe osteoarthritis pain, try the glucosamine-chondroitin combination for two to three months. If you find it eases your pain, it's reasonable to keep using it. If not, save your money.

As always, if you choose to take these or any other alternative preparations, be sure to inform your physician.

Acupuncture

Many people undergo acupuncture treatments to help relieve pain, including the pain of arthritis. Acupuncture, which involves the application of tiny, sterile needles to specific points in the skin, has been a staple of Chinese medicine for 2,000 years, and pain relief is one of its leading uses.

It may seem counterintuitive that needles could relieve pain, but the body appears to respond by releasing endorphins, a natural morphine-like chemical in the nervous system. An article in the *Cochrane Database of Systematic Reviews* looked at 16 studies involving nearly 3,500 people with osteoarthritis of the knee, hip, or hand. The studies compared acupuncture with sham acupuncture (in which needles were either inserted at incorrect points or didn't penetrate the skin), another treatment such as medication, or a waiting list control group. Compared with having fake acupuncture or being on a waiting list, real acupuncture offered small improvements in pain and function. But the benefit may have resulted from the placebo effect (the participants' expectations of improvement).

If you decide to try acupuncture, talk with your doctor first, and find a licensed acupuncturist. The typical cost of an acupuncture session ranges from

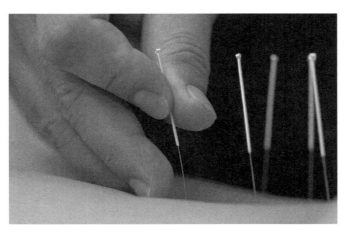

Acupuncture can help relieve pain, including the pain of arthritis, according to a number of studies. That may be because the body responds by releasing morphine-like chemicals called endorphins.

$65 to $125. It is not covered by Medicare, Medicaid, or most private insurers.

Massage

Many people with pain in their muscles and joints turn to massage therapy for relief. Some studies have shown that massage is safe and possibly effective. A review of seven studies that examined massage therapy for people with arthritis was published in 2017 in the *American Journal of Physical Medicine & Rehabilitation*. Together, the studies included 352 participants, and they found that people who received massage therapy had less pain and better ability to function in their daily lives than those who did not receive massage. However, the quality of the evidence was considered only low to moderate. Further research is needed.

Spinal manipulation

Chiropractors and osteopaths use spinal adjustments and other joint and soft-tissue manipulations to treat a variety of disorders of the muscles, bones, and nervous system. This therapy is often used for back pain, including pain from osteoarthritis in the spine. In one study, researchers randomly assigned 250 people with lower back pain due to osteoarthritis, degenerative disc disease, or both to receive either moist heat and chiropractic treatment or only moist heat. The people who got both therapies had less pain and a greater range of motion than those who did not receive the chiropractic treatment. But more research is needed to confirm the effectiveness of this approach. Doctors generally warn against rapid manipulation of the neck in people who have arthritis in the cervical spine.

On the horizon: Potential new treatments

Some of the following experimental approaches would have sounded like science fiction a generation ago, especially those that call upon the body's own regenerative capacities. But they are moving closer to becoming practical treatments—and some are already in use, even if they're not quite ready for prime time.

Platelet-rich plasma injections

Blood is made of several components, including red blood cells, white blood cells, plasma, and platelets. Platelets are of potential interest in treating osteoarthritis because they release proteins called growth factors, which have healing qualities. Platelet-rich plasma (PRP) therapy involves removing a small amount of blood from a person and spinning it in a device called a centrifuge to separate out the different components and increase the concentration of platelets. The platelet-rich plasma that results from this process is then injected into the site where healing is desired, such as in the knee joint of a person with knee osteoarthritis.

Some studies have found that PRP therapy is better than hyaluronate injections for people with minimal osteoarthritis. Young people benefited more than older ones. This technique is not used in routine practice but continues to be studied. It is expensive and not covered by insurance.

Stem cell injections

The body's stem cells have the ability to develop into any type of specialized cell, including chondrocytes, which produce cartilage. An experimental technique involves harvesting stem cells from a person's bone marrow, spinning them in a centrifuge to concentrate them, and then injecting the cells into the patient's affected joint. The idea is that these stem cells may transform into chondrocytes, thus restoring cartilage, reducing inflammation, and improving the ability to function.

Even though stem cell therapy is still in the experimental stages, clinics across the country already offer it. While this seems like a tempting solution to your joint problems, be aware that the science has not yet caught up with the hype, and you could even suffer harm. Clinics are allowed to perform the procedure because the FDA does not regulate treatments in which human cell and tissue products, such as blood, are taken from a person, minimally manipulated, and then injected back into the same person. However, the FDA is starting to scrutinize stem cell therapy more closely.

Stem cell therapy is quite expensive (for example, $2,000 to $5,000 per treatment) and, because it's unproven, it's not covered by insurance. Scientists are continuing to study stem cell treatment for osteoarthritis. If you want to try it, consider going to an academic medical center where researchers are testing the therapy, rather than trusting an independent clinic.

Chondrocyte grafting

In some people it may be possible to replace sections of degenerated cartilage. Chondrocyte grafting involves removing a small piece of cartilage, which is sent to a laboratory. The chondrocytes (cells that produce cartilage) are removed from the specimen and then processed to multiply in number. They are then injected into the joint, where they form new cartilage.

This technique appears to be most helpful for people with less severe defects in cartilage. People with severe osteoarthritis would require a large graft, which is not practical. ◆

Self-care strategies for coping with arthritis

The pain and stiffness of arthritis can make it difficult to perform the daily tasks most people take for granted, from putting on socks to cooking dinner. But taking good care of yourself—eating healthful foods, shedding pounds if you are overweight, strengthening muscles, and learning to move your joints safely—can help you relieve your pain, improve daily functioning, and cope with difficult emotions, no matter what form of arthritis you have. In addition, you may find relief by trying physical therapy (see "Physical and occupational therapy," page 16) or complementary therapies, such as acupuncture and massage (see "Complementary therapies," page 23). The American College of Rheumatology recommends not only medication but also nondrug treatments for people with osteoarthritis of the hip and knee.

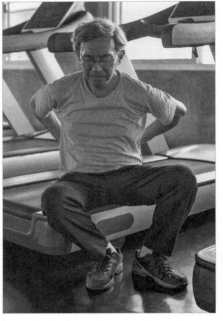

It can be hard to make yourself exercise if you have joint pain. But a lack of exercise may only lead to more pain and stiffness.

Following are some do-it-yourself strategies and therapies that can make coping with arthritis a little easier.

Heat therapy

In the 19th and early 20th centuries, wealthy Europeans embraced hydrotherapy (warm baths) and sought cures at exotic spas for real and imagined ailments. Most resorts claimed that the health benefits were from minerals in the water. However, the therapeutic value probably lay mostly in the water's temperature. Heat raises the pain threshold and relaxes muscles. Heat is particularly helpful for joints that are stiff.

Hydrotherapy can be used at home. A hot tub or a bathtub equipped with water jets can closely duplicate the warm-water massage of whirlpool baths used by physical therapists. For most people, the bathtub works nearly as well as a whirlpool. Soaking for 15 to 20 minutes in a warm bath exposes the body to warmth and allows the weight-bearing muscles to relax.

A warm shower can also relieve the stiffness of arthritis. You can upgrade your shower with an adjustable shower-head massager that's inexpensive and easy to install. It should deliver a steady, fine spray or a pulsing stream, usually with a few options in between.

Therapists also recommend taking a warm shower or bath before exercising to relax joints and muscles. Dress warmly after a shower or bath to prolong the benefit.

A heating pad is another good idea, but keep in mind that moist heat penetrates more deeply. Although you can purchase hot packs and moist/dry heating pads, a homemade hot pack works just as well. Heat a damp folded towel in a microwave oven (usually for about 20 to 60 seconds, depending on the oven and the towel's thickness) or in an oven set at 300° F (for five to 10 minutes—again, this depends on the oven and towel thickness). To prevent burns, always test the heated towel on the inside of your arm before applying it to a joint: it should feel comfortably warm, not hot. To be extra safe, wrap the heated, moist towel in a thin, dry one before placing it on the skin.

Another way to warm up stiff painful hands and feet is a paraffin bath. Paraffin bath kits are available for home use and are also used by physical therapists. You dip your hands or feet into wax melted in an electric appliance that maintains a safe temperature. After the wax hardens, the treated area is wrapped in a plastic sheet and blanket to retain the heat. Treatments generally take about 20 minutes, after which the wax is peeled off. Before using a home paraffin kit, talk with your physical therapist for recommendations and cautions.

Cold therapy

When it comes to osteoarthritis, cold has painkilling effects that are similar to those of heat. Gel-filled cold packs are inexpensive and available in different sizes and shapes. Keep two or more in the freezer so you'll have cold therapy available instantly. Ice chips in a plastic bag also work well. However, you should never apply ice directly to bare skin; put a thin towel in between. Cold packs should be applied for 15 to 20 minutes and can be reapplied hourly or as needed. Coolant sprays, available from pharmacies, may also be used. Cooling is a temporary measure to relieve pain; too much may induce muscle stiffness and painful circulatory disturbances.

Exercise

Even the healthiest people find it difficult to stick with an exercise regimen. But those with arthritis commonly discover that if they don't exercise regularly, they'll pay the price in pain, stiffness, and fatigue. Regular exercise not only helps maintain joint function, but also relieves stiffness and decreases pain and fatigue. Feeling tired may be partly the result of inflammation and medications, but it's also caused by muscle weakness and poor stamina.

Getting regular exercise doesn't have to be overly burdensome. Walking counts as exercise, as long as you do enough of it. Walking is a weight-bearing exercise, which is especially important for joints like the knee, hip, and ankle. Cartilage needs nourishment, which it gets from synovial fluid. Some form of compression is required for synovial fluid to circulate across the whole joint. With every step you take, synovial fluid provides nutrients to cartilage, which may help to slow down deterioration.

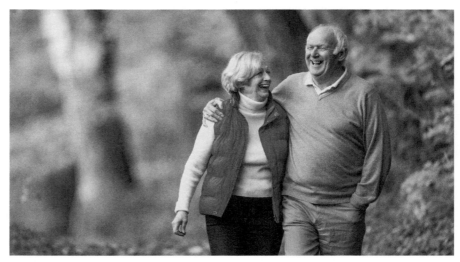

© SolStock | Getty Images

Walking may help slow deterioration in the knees and hips. This may be because pressure from walking forces synovial fluid to circulate across the joints, providing nutrition to cartilage.

If you've been relatively inactive, start a walking program slowly. Gradually build up to 30 minutes a day, at least five days a week. The 30 minutes can be broken up into 10-minute segments, and all walking counts, whether it's around the house, down the street, or on a treadmill. Start at a moderate pace, but aim to build up to a brisk walk (about 2.5 to 3.5 mph).

These tips may also help:

- Schedule walks for times of the day when you are least likely to experience pain.
- Before walking, apply heat. After walking, cold packs may be helpful.
- Warm up by marching in place or walking at a slower pace than normal.

Many electronic devices are on the market to help you count steps. These devices can help get you motivated. If you think that will help, consider starting with an inexpensive pedometer before investing in a more expensive fitness tracker that has additional functions, like counting calories and tracking sleep. The goal often cited is 10,000 steps a day, but you don't necessarily have to walk that much to see benefits. A study published in *Arthritis Care & Research* found that people with knee osteoarthritis benefited from walking just 6,000 steps or more a day. After two years, they had less limitation in physical functioning.

If you want go beyond walking, try the types of exercise that are most helpful for people with osteoarthritis. A review of numerous studies found that strength training, water-based exercises, and balance therapy were the most helpful for reducing pain and improving function.

Following are brief descriptions of various forms of exercise, including structured exercise programs (most of which are offered by local Arthritis Foundation chapters), that provide potential benefits for people with arthritis.

Land-based programs. These include community-based group

Four exercise goals

Structured exercise programs commonly emphasize one or more of these goals. You can also work with your physician or physical therapist to develop your own exercise program that addresses them all.

1 **Increase range of motion.** Stretches and range-of-motion exercises aim to improve the mobility and flexibility of your joints. To increase your range of motion, move a joint as far as it can go and then try to push a little farther. These exercises can be done any time, even when your joints are painful, as long as you do them gently. For several examples of range-of-motion exercises you can do at home, see Figure 9, page 30.

2 **Strengthen your muscles.** An excellent way to provide aching joints with more support is to strengthen the muscles surrounding them. Strengthening exercises use resistance to build muscles. You can use your own body weight as resistance. One example: Sit in a chair. Now lean forward and stand by pushing up with your thigh muscles (try to use your arms only for balance). Stand a moment, then sit back down, using your thigh muscles. This simple exercise will help ease the strain on your knees by building up these muscles. Research has shown that strengthening the thigh muscles is just as effective as aerobic exercise or NSAIDs for reducing pain and disability. Furthermore, research suggests that strengthening these muscles might even slow the narrowing of the joint space in people with arthritis of the knee.

3 **Build endurance.** Aerobic activities such as walking, swimming, and bicycling can build your heart and lung function, which in turn increases endurance and overall health. Movement also helps lubricate joints. However, you should avoid high-impact activities such as jogging.

4 **Improve balance.** Physical therapists often include better balance in their lists of goals. This is important because people with osteoarthritis, especially in the knees, are at increased risk of falling. There are simple ways to work on balance. For example, stand with your weight on both feet. Then try lifting one foot while you balance on the other foot for five seconds. Repeat on the other side. (You might want to stand by a chair that you can grab on to just in case.) Over time, see if you can work your way up to 30 seconds. Yoga and tai chi—which involve slow, controlled movements or positions that are held for a set period—are also good for balance.

classes led by health or fitness professionals with specialized training in instructing people with arthritis. These programs typically include some combination of a warm-up routine and several standard exercise goals (see "Four exercise goals," page 28), plus specialized activities to enhance body awareness, balance, and coordination. Examples include Fit and Strong, a program targeted to older adults with osteoarthritis; the Arthritis Foundation's Exercise Program (AFEP); and its Walk with Ease program. Studies have found that people with arthritis in their hips, legs, and feet who took Fit and Strong classes were able to exercise longer, felt more confident about their ability to exercise, and reported less joint stiffness compared with those in a control group. Many of the benefits lasted between six and 12 months. Those attending AFEP classes for eight weeks had less pain, stiffness, and fatigue, and these improvements persisted at least six months, as well. In one study, people who completed the Walk with Ease program (which also teaches participants about managing their arthritis) had more confidence, less depression, and less pain, compared with participants who attended classes that focused only on pain management.

Water-based programs. Also known as aquatic or pool therapy, these group classes are done in warm water and feature a variety of exercises, including range-of-

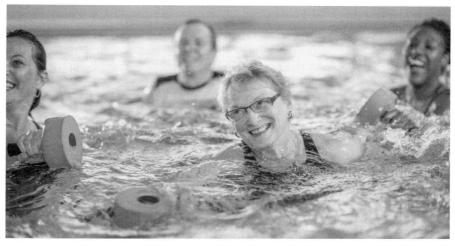

Exercise helps relieve osteoarthritis pain by building the muscles that support aching joints and by loosening stiff muscles. Water-based exercise programs are particularly good for people with arthritis, since the water helps support some of your weight.

motion exercises and aerobics. Exercising in water has many benefits for people with arthritis. For example, the buoyancy of the water supports some of your weight. The deeper you go, the more weight is supported. At waist level, the water supports about 50% of your weight, and in water up to your chest, it is about 75%. Studies show that exercising in water lessens arthritis pain and boosts fitness.

Strength and resistance training. This form of exercise, which uses equipment such as weight machines, free weights, and resistance bands or tubing, strengthens not only your muscles but also your bones and cardiovascular system. Resistance training improves muscle strength, physical functioning, and pain. One Japanese study compared people with knee osteoarthritis who either took NSAIDs or did twice-daily knee extension exercises to strengthen

their quadriceps (the muscles on the front of the thigh). At the end of the eight-week study, both groups had less pain and stiffness, as well as improved functioning and quality of life.

Tai chi. With origins in Chinese martial arts, this low-impact, slow-motion exercise also emphasizes breathing and mental focus. It involves moving continuously through a series of motions named for animal actions—for example, "white crane spreads its wings"— or martial arts moves, such as "box both ears." The movements are usually circular and never forced, the muscles are relaxed rather than tensed, the joints are not fully extended or bent, and connective tissues are not stretched.

A number of small studies suggest tai chi helps people with different forms of arthritis, mainly by increasing flexibility and improving muscle strength in the lower body,

Figure 9: Range-of-motion exercises for arthritis

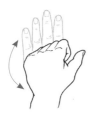

Hand Open your hand, holding the fingers straight. Bend the middle finger joints. Next, touch your fingertips to the top of your palm. Open your hand. Repeat 10 times with each hand.

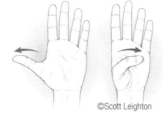

Next, reach your thumb across your hand to touch the base of your little finger. Stretch your thumb back out. Repeat 10 times.

©Scott Leighton

Shoulder Lie on your back with your hands at your sides. Raise one arm slowly over your head, keeping your arm close to your ear and your elbow straight. Return your arm to your side. Repeat with the other arm. Repeat 10 times.

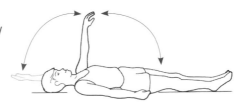

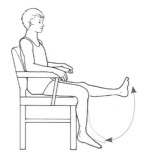

Knee Sit in a chair that is high enough for you to swing your legs. Keep your thighs on the seat and straighten out one leg. Hold for a few seconds. Then bend your knee and bring your foot as far back as possible. Repeat with the other leg. Repeat 10 times.

Hip Lie on your back, legs straight and about 6 inches apart. Point your toes toward the ceiling. Slide one leg out to the side and then back to its original position. Try to keep your toes pointed up the whole time. Repeat 10 times with each leg.

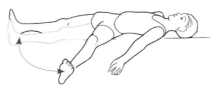

All illustrations ©Harriet Greenfield (except upper right)

as well as aiding gait and balance. The Arthritis Foundation developed a standardized form of tai chi designed specifically for people with arthritis. Based on Sun-style tai chi, one of the discipline's five major recognized styles, it includes agile steps and a high stance (meaning the legs bend only slightly).

Yoga. There is growing evidence that yoga may help with the pain and stiffness of osteoarthritis. A review published in the *American Journal of Physical Medicine & Rehabilitation*, which examined results from 12 studies, found that yoga reduced pain, stiffness, and swelling in people with osteoarthritis.

Yoga sessions typically last from 45 to 90 minutes, but you can also benefit from practicing yoga at home for 10 to 20 minutes a few times a week. DVDs with yoga instruction are widely available. A session generally begins with breathing exercises to relax the body and help free the mind of worries and distractions. Breathing deeply through the nose is a vital component of yoga. The session then proceeds through a series of seated, standing, and lying postures (asanas), which you may be instructed to hold for a few seconds to minutes. Holding the body correctly in the various postures and breathing into them to stretch farther is important, but you should never push your body farther than it wishes to go, and you should stop if you feel any pain. The sessions typically end with meditation.

Yoga postures can be modified to accommodate your strength and experience, as well as any health conditions. Be sure to tell your instructor about osteoarthritis and any other health problems you have, so he or she can warn you against certain positions that may aggravate your pain and suggest alternatives or appropriate modifications.

You can find classes offering several different forms of yoga. Look for one that is at your level and caters to your needs. This may be a beginning class or a chair yoga class. For osteoarthritis, you should probably avoid the more strenuous forms of yoga, such as Ashtanga or power yoga, which may aggravate already damaged joints. Although some studies have found Iyengar yoga to be helpful for people with arthritis, others have found that this form of yoga, where static postures are held for longer periods of time, can be painful. A gentle Vinyasa or flow class may be less painful. Check with your doctor before trying a rigorous form of yoga or one performed in a very hot room.

Balance exercises. Stiff, sore joints hamper movement. If your ankles or knees are arthritic, it's hard to bend them, which affects your ability to balance and react when you trip. Tai chi and some yoga poses help with balance. There also are exercises specifically designed to improve balance that can be safely performed, even if your balance is shaky. You can find many examples of these in another Harvard Special Health Report, *Better Balance: Simple exercises to improve stability and prevent falls* (see "Resources," page 52).

A stiff neck can also affect balance, by causing you to move your upper body instead of just your head to look behind you. (For an exercise to relieve neck stiffness, see Figure 10, at right.)

Joint protection strategies

When you have arthritis, it's important to pay attention to your body's signals. Overuse of arthritic joints can lead to pain, swelling, and additional joint damage. A

physical or occupational therapist can teach you how to protect your joints, accomplish daily tasks more easily, and adapt to lifestyle disruptions. Many of these strategies are simple common sense.

Keep moving. Avoid holding one position for too long. When working at a desk, for example, get up and stretch every 15 minutes. Do the same while sitting at home reading or watching television.

Avoid stressing your joints. Avoid positions or movements that put extra stress on joints. For example, opening a tight lid can be

difficult if you have hand arthritis. One solution is to set the jar on a cloth, lean on the jar with your palm, and turn the lid using a shoulder motion. Better yet, purchase a wall-mounted jar opener that grips the lid, leaving both hands free to turn the jar.

Discover your strength. Use your strongest joints and muscles. To protect finger and wrist joints, push open heavy doors with the side of the arm or shoulder. To reduce hip or knee stress on stairs, lead with the stronger leg going up and the weaker leg going down.

Figure 10: An exercise to relieve neck pain

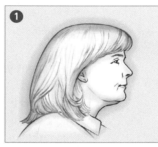
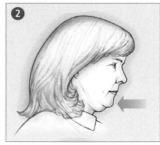
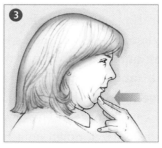

Here is a simple, gentle exercise to do when moderate neck pain first strikes. For severe pain, contact your health care provider immediately.

1. Sit in a neutral position, holding your head in a normal resting position.

2. Next, slowly glide your head backward, tucking your chin in until you have pulled your head and chin as far back as they will go. Keep your head level and do not tilt or nod your head. Pull in gently for three to five seconds, then release. Repeat 10 times.

3. For a stronger stretch, gently apply pressure to your chin with your fingers and release. Repeat every two hours as needed.

If this exercise increases your pain, try it lying down on your back. Tuck your chin in and make a double chin. Hold for a second or two and release (your head never leaves the pillow). If pain increases or you develop numbness or tingling, stop and contact your doctor.

Helpful gadgets

Simple gadgets and devices can sometimes make it easier to perform daily activities, such as cooking, gardening, or even getting dressed. For example, people with limited movement might have an easier time using long-handled hooks when putting on socks and long-handled shoehorns for shoes. Also helpful are shoes that slip on or fasten with Velcro, pre-tied neckties, and garments with Velcro fasteners, zippers, or hooks and eyes instead of buttons. For other tasks, long-handled grippers are designed to grasp and retrieve out-of-reach objects. Rubber grips are available to help you get a better hold on faucets, pens, toothbrushes, and silverware. Ergonomic tools with long necks and comfortable grips are also useful. Pharmacies, medical supply stores, and online vendors stock a variety of aids for people with arthritis. The following will give you an idea of the broad array of tools available.

In the kitchen

- mini chopper
- electric can opener
- wall-mounted jar opener
- small, nonskid gripper mats to increase traction when opening jars and to place under bowls and other items to prevent slippage
- utensils with built-up, padded handles
- loop or spring-loaded scissors
- cheese slicer
- bottle brush, for washing cups and glasses
- cookbook stand

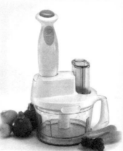

Mini chopper

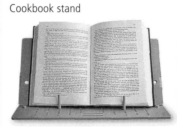

Cookbook stand

In the bathroom

- electric toothbrush
- dental floss holder
- electric razor
- soap-on-a-rope or mitts to hold soap in the shower
- brushes or combs with long handles
- raised toilet seat
- long-handled brush to clean the bathtub

In the yard and garden

- kneeler and seat
- ergonomic tools (with long necks and comfortable grips)
- motor-driven hose reel
- angled shovel
- hose caddy
- raised garden beds
- low-maintenance plants
- carpenter's apron with several pockets for carrying frequently used tools

Throughout your home and car

- key turners
- doorknob turners
- light switch adapters
- lightweight vacuum cleaner
- scissors with padded handles or swivel blades (loop or spring-loaded)
- rollerball or gel pens, pencils with padded grips

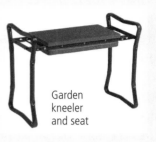

Garden kneeler and seat

Light switch adapter

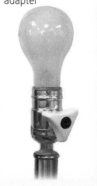

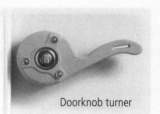

Key turner

Doorknob turner

Plan ahead. Simplify your life as much as possible. Eliminate unnecessary activities. (For example, save yourself work by buying clothing that doesn't need ironing.) Organize work and storage areas, and place frequently used items within easy reach. Keep duplicate household items in several locations; for example, stock the kitchen and all bathrooms with cleaning supplies.

Use labor-saving items and adaptive aids. In the kitchen, use electric can openers and mixers. In the bathroom, cut down on scrubbing by using automatic toilet bowl cleaners and, in showers or tubs, spray-on mildew remover. Other devices can help you avoid unnecessary bending, stooping, or reaching (see "Helpful gadgets," above).

Make home modifications. Using casters on furniture can make housecleaning easier. A grab bar mounted over the tub is a necessity for many people, as is a suction mat in the tub to prevent falls. Putting a bathing stool in the tub or shower is a good idea for people who have arthritis in the legs.

Ask for help. Maintaining independence is essential to self-esteem, but independence at all costs is a recipe for disaster. Achieve a balance by educating family members and friends about arthritis and the limitations it imposes and enlisting their support. Give them guidance by asking for help with specific tasks.

Healthy eating

There is no definitive evidence that any particular foods contribute to osteoarthritis pain or help to treat it. Yet, diet is important, especially if you are overweight. Excess pounds increase the stress on your joints, and obesity is a known risk factor for hand and knee osteoarthritis. To shed pounds or keep them off, exercise regularly and eat a healthy diet. This means eating plenty of vegetables, fruits, legumes, and whole grains. At the same time, minimize processed foods, which tend to be high in salt, fat, and sugar. Unprocessed or minimally processed foods contain fewer calories and more fiber, so you'll feel fuller longer.

Scientists have been studying whether foods with anti-inflammatory properties can help, since the wear and tear of osteoarthri-

tis can be accompanied by mild inflammation in joints. Some evidence suggests that omega-3 fats, found in cold-water fish such as salmon, herring, sardines, and mackerel, may be beneficial. The anti-inflammatory spice turmeric (an ingredient in curry) has also been tested for its ability to reduce the pain and tenderness of arthritis (both osteoarthritis and rheumatoid arthritis). Early results have shown promise, but larger and longer-term studies are needed.

Coping with your emotions

People with arthritis often worry about the possibility of losing mobility, being unable to work, or growing dependent on others. But only a very small percentage of people with arthritis ever become severely disabled. Still, the emotional burdens of arthritis are considerable and may result in stress, anxiety, and depression.

Because living with chronic arthritis can be difficult, many physicians use questionnaires to

---

Choosing shoes: What not to wear

Many types of arthritis affect the feet, so choosing a comfortable shoe is key. People with osteoarthritis may develop osteophytes at the base of their big toes. These abnormal bone growths can contribute to the joint enlargement and toe pain associated with bunions.

Clearly, pointy-toed shoes and high heels—which crowd the toes and put undue pressure on them—are not a good idea. High heels are also hard on the knees. Experts say that even a modest 1.5-inch heel increases pressure in two common sites for osteoarthritis damage: the joint beneath the undersurface of the kneecap (the patellofemoral compartment) and the joint surfaces on the inner side of the knee (the medial compartment).

Instead, choose a fairly flat shoe—low heels, no higher than three-quarters of an inch, are best. Also, select shoes with only a small amount of arch support, thereby allowing the foot to strike the ground and move forward as naturally as possible. Good choices for people with toe problems include shoes with a wide toe box, such as square-toed boots. Rheumatologists also recommend running shoes because they're lightweight and typically have good support for the foot in general, with some support (but not too much) in the arch and padding both in the soles and around the ankles.

To add more cushioning, you can purchase foot orthotics over the counter. Brands include Powerstep, Superfeet, and Spenco. Look for styles with no-tie shoelaces or Velcro fasteners, especially if you have hand arthritis.

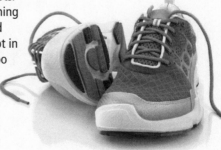

Running shoes, with their padding and support, can make good shoes for everyday use.

assess a person's psychological function. Depression and anxiety are of particular concern, as these disorders are twice as common among people with arthritis than people without it.

Your doctor may also ask questions about what type of family and social support you have available, to determine whether you need additional help. For example, if you live alone and have trouble walking, your doctor may refer you to a social worker who can help arrange for someone to handle shopping and other chores. If you show signs of depression or anxiety, you may be referred to a psychiatrist.

Depression is common in people with chronic diseases of all kinds. Some arthritis specialists have assumed that depression is directly related to the amount of pain and the number of swollen joints a person has, but this isn't always the case. While some people equate a large number of swollen joints with severe disability, those whose favorite pastime is reading or spending time with family might not consider themselves disabled. However, a relatively slight impairment in hand mobility could be devastating for a pianist or artist, and could have a profound emotional impact. Diagnosing and treating depression can be challenging because its symptoms differ from person to person. But effective medications are available, and they often work best in combination with counseling or psychotherapy. A form of counseling called cognitive behavioral therapy involves changing people's behaviors by changing their thinking.

Sexual intimacy

Arthritis may interfere with sexual intimacy, especially when the hips, knees, or spine are involved. However, even people with severe arthritis can enjoy an active sex life. A flexible attitude often compensates quite well for having a less-than-flexible body. For example, couples might experiment with different positions to find the one most comfortable for intercourse; people with hip, knee, or spine arthritis often find it most comfortable when both parties lie on their side. There are also other mutually gratifying sexual activities besides intercourse.

Many people find that taking a pain reliever an hour before sex or having a warm shower lessens muscle and joint stiffness. Rescheduling sexual activity may also help; afternoons may be better if pain and fatigue are worse in the mornings or evenings. But arthritis needn't hold you back. ◗

Surgical treatment of osteoarthritis

Sometimes people need surgery to relieve extremely painful or badly misaligned joints. The option your doctor recommends will depend on your age, activity level, and overall health. Surgical options are usually recommended only when drug therapies and other strategies no longer work and osteoarthritis significantly limits daily activities.

Arthroscopy

As a consequence of osteoarthritis, tiny pieces of cartilage can break off and float around in the joint space. Other debris can also accumulate. And in the knee joint, the menisci are susceptible to tearing. A meniscus is a C-shaped piece of cartilage located in the knee joint where the thighbone meets the shin bone. There are two of them in each knee, one on each side (see Figure 4, page 8). Small meniscal tears can occur over time as you age. A meniscus can also tear suddenly from an injury.

It's long been thought that cleaning out the debris at the joint (called debridement) and repairing torn menisci should help with pain relief. To accomplish this, surgeons perform arthroscopic surgery. Arthroscopy is considered minor surgery because the incisions are small and the procedure generally does not require an overnight stay in the hospital. To do the procedure, the surgeon inserts an arthroscope—an instrument with a tiny light and a camera on its tip—into the joint through a small incision. A variety of surgical attachments can be passed through the arthroscope or inserted separately through additional small incisions. Using these tools, the surgeon removes torn cartilage, debris, and loose material.

While this is a common procedure, several studies have questioned the usefulness of it for most cases of osteoarthritis. A study published in the journal *BMJ* reviewed nine studies that assessed the benefits of using arthroscopic surgery to debride or partially remove a torn meniscus in middle-aged and older

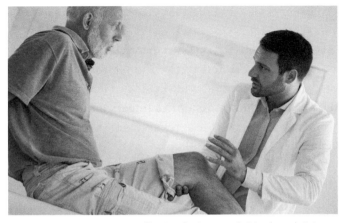

Arthroscopic surgery is not effective for knee arthritis, though it is useful for certain other problems, like a torn meniscus. For severe osteoarthritis of the knee, total knee replacement is a better option.

adults with knee pain. The researchers found that there was a small improvement in the first three to six months after the procedure. However, the benefit disappeared within two years. Arthroscopic surgery on the knee also had no effect on improving physical functioning. So, arthroscopy as a means for treating osteoarthritis might not be helpful.

This does not mean that arthroscopic surgery never has a role in treatment. For example, people who have a torn meniscus from a sudden injury or a large piece of cartilage floating in the joint space can benefit from the procedure.

Alternatives to joint replacement

For a badly damaged knee or hip, joint replacement (see page 36) is regarded as the definitive treatment. However, it is generally considered a last resort and is not right for everyone. Here are some other surgical options.

Realignment

Surgery can be performed to realign bones that are no longer correctly lined up as a result of osteoarthritis.

© gilaxia | Getty Images

In the case of knee osteoarthritis, for example, the surgeon reshapes the tibia (shin bone) and femur (thighbone) to improve the alignment of the knee joint. This may be an alternative to joint replacement for people who are young and active and not yet candidates for an implant that lasts only 15 to 20 years.

Fusion

Another possibility involves permanently fusing two bones at the affected joint. This is an option when arthritis occurs in parts of the body such as the wrist, ankle, and small joints of the fingers and toes, where joint replacement is less reliable and performed less often.

Hip resurfacing

Hip resurfacing may offer an attractive alternative to traditional hip replacement, especially for younger and more active people. It preserves more bone and may allow for greater mobility. Instead of removing the head of the femur and replacing it with an artificial ball, the surgeon reshapes the head and places a metal cap over it, which fits into a metal lining in the socket. Resurfacing uses a bigger ball, which some surgeons say makes dislocation less likely and gives the joint the ability to handle greater stress. Because resurfacing preserves the neck and part of the head of the thighbone, it also makes it easier and less complicated to have a traditional hip replacement in the future when the resurfacing wears out, compared with redoing a failed total hip replacement.

Hip resurfacing was first tried in the 1970s, but it fell out of favor because of problems with the polyethylene parts used at the time. Since then, a newer generation of metal-on-metal caps and socket linings has been approved by the FDA. Still, the procedure has not been studied as extensively or for as long as hip replacement, and people with hip resurfacing seem to be more likely to have complications, including fractures of the upper portion of the thighbone, compared with those who have had conventional hip replacement. These complications appear to be most common in people with smaller bones, including women. Studies going back 10 years suggest that hip resurfacing offers the best benefit-to-risk ratio for men under age 60 who need a total hip replacement and would like to remain active.

Joint replacement

Doctors recommend joint replacement in cases of severe osteoarthritis in which the joint shows significant deterioration. This surgery is most often recommended for osteoarthritis of the knee or hip, because severe disease of these joints can impede movement. In fact, knee replacement and hip replacement are among the most common elective surgeries in the United States, with more than 680,000 total knee replacements and over 370,000 total hip replacements performed each year.

Success rates for these procedures are high, at over 90%, but it is important to have realistic expectations. You probably won't regain the function you had in your youth. A new hip or knee, however, should allow you to engage in normal activities again and function much better. The major consistent benefit of joint replacement is substantial relief from pain. To maximize the chances of good results, it's important to participate in physical therapy before and after surgery.

A replaced joint will last an average of 15 to 20 years. Surgeons may encourage young, physically active people to delay joint replacement because artificial joints may need to be replaced after a decade or two. The younger the person, the greater the chances that surgery will need to be repeated later on—and repeat surgery is more difficult because there is less bone to work with after removing the first implant.

However, it's possible to wait too long before getting a joint replacement. Severe arthritis can cause structural deformities in the joint that may not be possible to correct with joint replacement. As a result, waiting until joint problems have severely limited your function may lessen the benefit you get from knee or hip replacement (see "When is it time?" on page 37).

Knee implants

For knee replacement, the surgeon fits a metal implant over the end of the thighbone and another one over the shin bone where the two bones meet (see Figure 11, page 38). A thick piece of plastic

When is it time? Making the decision to have a joint replacement

If the pain and limitations of osteoarthritis are significantly interfering with your life, talk with your doctor about whether replacing your knee or hip joint is a good solution. Joint replacement is an elective procedure, and it is not an option for everyone. The ideal candidate is in good general health and not overweight. The average age of people undergoing joint replacement has been declining. For total knee replacement, it is 66, and for total hip replacement it is 65. The decision to have joint replacement is ultimately up to you and your physician. Together, you must weigh the benefits and risks.

You may want to consider joint replacement if one or more of the following statements apply to you:

- You are unable to complete normal daily tasks without help.
- You have significant pain daily.
- Pain keeps you awake at night despite the use of medications.
- Nonsurgical approaches—such as medications, the use of a cane, and diligent physical therapy—have not relieved your pain.
- Less complicated surgical procedures are unlikely to help.
- Pain keeps you from walking or bending over.
- Pain doesn't stop when you rest.
- You can't bend or straighten your knee, or your hip is so stiff that you can't lift your leg.
- You are suffering severe side effects from the medications for your joint symptoms.
- X-rays show advanced arthritis.

Joint replacement is generally not an option for people with any of the following problems:

- systemic infection or infection in the damaged knee or hip
- leg circulation so poor that it will interfere with healing
- severely damaged or nonworking muscles or ligaments that do not properly support the knee joint
- damaged nerves in the legs
- neuromuscular disease such as multiple sclerosis, Parkinson's disease, or stroke
- allergy to metal or plastic
- medical illness that makes any major surgery risky.

Like any major operation, joint replacement surgery carries the risk of complications. For example, there is a small chance that you may have an adverse reaction to the anesthesia, develop a blood clot, contract an infection, or suffer other complications that are specific to knee and hip replacement (see "Possible complications of joint replacement," page 40).

---

mounted onto the shin implant serves the same purpose as natural cartilage, allowing for smooth flowing movement. The kneecap is fitted with a small metal and plastic disc.

There are many brands and designs of knee implants to choose from, depending on your age, weight, activity level, and health. The most common type is called a fixed-bearing knee prosthesis. The tibial component of the prosthesis is topped with a flat metal piece that securely holds a polyethylene (plastic) insert. When the knee is in motion, the femoral component glides across the polyethylene. Another type of implant is a rotating-platform knee prosthesis, in which the polyethylene insert can rotate slightly, theoretically lessening stress and wear on the implant and improving movement.

If damage to the cartilage is limited to one of the two bumps (condyles) on the end of the thighbone, a partial knee replacement may be performed. This is a less extensive procedure with a shorter hospital stay and quicker recovery. But it lasts only about 10 years, on average, compared with 15 to 20 years for total knee replacement.

Hip implants

There are dozens of hip implant models. The decision on which one to use depends on a person's weight, bone quality, age, occupation, and activity level, as well as the surgeon's experience with particular brands and models.

Hip implants have two parts: a socket and a ball mounted on a long stem (see Figure 12, page 39). The components are a combination of hard polished metal (generally titanium-based or cobalt-chromium-based alloy), hard ceramic, or tough, slick plastic called polyethylene. There are currently four types of hip implants:

- **Metal on polyethylene:** The ball is made of metal and the socket is made of polyethylene (plastic) or has a plastic lining.

- **Ceramic on polyethylene:** The ball is made of ceramic and the socket is made of polyethylene or has a plastic lining.
- **Ceramic on ceramic:** The ball is made of ceramic and the socket has a ceramic lining.
- **Ceramic on metal:** The ball is made of ceramic and the socket has a metal lining.

Metal-on-metal hip implants have fallen out of favor because of problems with their design. As the metal ball and metal cup slide against each other, tiny metal particles can wear off and enter the space around the implant. In many cases, this resulted in loosening of the implant, requiring a second surgery. If you have a metal-on-metal device that was implanted earlier, this does not mean you necessarily have to undergo surgery to replace it. As long as it continues to function without problems, you should simply follow up with your surgeon as often as he or she recommends (usually every one to two years). If you develop new

---

Figure 11: Total knee replacement

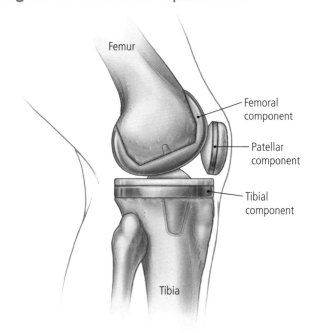

The surgeon first cuts away thin slices of bone with damaged cartilage from the end of the femur (thighbone) and the top of the tibia (shin bone), making sure that the bones are cut to precisely fit the shape of the replacement pieces. The artificial joint is attached to the bones with cement or screws. A small plastic piece goes on the back of the kneecap (patella) to ride smoothly over the other parts of the artificial joint when you bend your knee.

---

or significantly worsening symptoms, such as hip or groin pain, swelling, numbness, noise (popping, grinding, clicking, or squeaking of your hip), or a change in your ability to walk, don't wait for your regular follow-up appointment, but contact your surgeon to discuss your options.

Minimally invasive techniques

Some surgeons have special training to use minimally invasive techniques for hip or knee replacement surgery. This means that the surgery is performed by making smaller incisions and using smaller instruments. The goals are to reduce soft-tissue injury and blood loss and to speed recovery. So far, results have been promising, at least among young, active individuals who were treated in hospitals that perform a large number of these procedures. But whether the overall results are better than (or even comparable to) traditional joint replacement surgery for the general public is not clear, especially considering that even traditional joint replacement is now often done with a smaller incision than in the past.

Two joints at the same time

Some people have significant osteoarthritic pain in both knees or both hips and want to have joint replacement on both sides. This usually is done in two separate surgeries several months apart, but it is also possible to have both joints replaced at the same time (simultaneous replacement). The benefits of simultaneous replacement are a single operation and one rehabilitation. However, having simultaneous replacement increases the risk of some complications. For example, with simultaneous replacement there is a slightly increased risk for blood clots. And, while you only have to go through rehabilitation once rather than twice, it takes longer when both joints are replaced at the same time.

Not all surgeons will perform simultaneous replacement. If they do, they usually consider it only for people at low risk for possible complications.

Preparing for joint replacement

Because joint replacement for osteoarthritis is elective surgery, it will be scheduled weeks or even months ahead of time. In the period leading up to the surgery, you may be asked to take some steps to ensure a successful outcome. For example, if you are overweight you may be advised to lose some pounds, because excess weight can lead to postsurgical complications. If you smoke, try to quit, as smoking affects blood flow and may slow recovery.

Your surgeon may recommend a presurgical physical therapy program (often called prehabilitation, or prehab). This is helpful because muscles surrounding a joint that's so painful it requires replacing may have atrophied somewhat from decreased use. Improving strength and endurance in the joint before replacement may mean less pain after the surgery and may speed recovery during postsurgical rehabilitation. A physical therapist can guide you through an appropriate exercise regimen that builds strength without putting too much stress on an extremely painful joint. The physical therapist will also teach you about postsurgical exercises so you will be prepared for what will happen after the surgery.

Recovering from joint replacement

Postoperative recovery will vary depending on your health and age. You'll be in the hospital for about two to three days. But this doesn't mean you'll just be lying in bed. A nurse or physical therapist is likely to get you up and walking a short distance with crutches or a walker a day or two after surgery. You will also be given exercises to perform.

Before you can safely return home, you are usually expected to be able to do the following: get in and out of bed, walk with crutches or a walker, step on and off a curb, climb the same number of steps you must negotiate at home, perform your rehab exercises, and show you can carry out necessary tasks with little or no assistance. If you had knee replacement, you should be able to straighten your knee and bend it 90°. If you are unable to do these things or need extra nursing care, you may be discharged temporarily to a rehabilitation facility.

While you are in the hospital recovering from the surgery, your pain will be controlled with powerful pain medications if needed. Advances in anesthesia, including the use of regional anesthesia (so you can

Figure 12: Hip replacement surgery

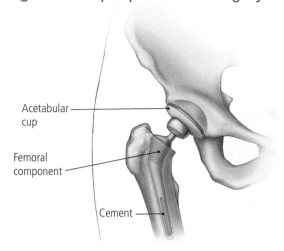

Acetabular cup

Femoral component

Cement

When rough and damaged cartilage prevents the bones of the hip from moving smoothly, an orthopedic surgeon can install an artificial joint with two parts. The head of the femur (thighbone) is replaced with an artificial ball with a long stem that fits down inside the femur. An artificial cup, called the acetabular cup, fits inside the hip socket. The two pieces fit smoothly together to restore comfortable ball-in-socket movement.

alert the doctor to pain sooner, rather than after you wake up), have resulted in better pain control after surgery and less need for strong opioid (narcotic) medications. The amount of pain you will experience once you return home is hard to predict. Some people have very little pain and get relief from ordinary nonprescription pain relievers. Others have more severe pain and need something stronger.

It's not always clear why a person may experience exceptional pain. It can be a matter of perception—people's thresholds for pain vary tremendously. In other cases, there may be an underlying problem causing the pain, such as an inflamed tendon or an infection. The important thing to remember is that you should never suffer in silence. If your pain level is unacceptable, call your surgeon or primary care physician. If there's an underlying cause, he or she can address it. For example, pain caused by an inflamed tendon can be alleviated with a steroid shot, and infections can be cured with antibiotics (or, on occasion, additional surgery).

If there is no direct cause, the doctor can prescribe a more powerful medication, such as oxycodone (OxyContin, Percocet). This drug is an opioid medication and is tightly regulated because of its potential for abuse.

Rehabilitation after joint replacement

Because joint replacement is an elective surgery, you will have time before the procedure to plan for the recovery period afterward. It can take several months to return to normal functioning. During this time, you will gradually improve and regain strength and agility in the joint. But be aware that you will have limited mobility at first.

To ease the recovery, plan ahead. Set up an area in your home in which you'll spend most of your time. Your phone, remote control, reading materials, medications, and water should be within easy reach. Remove scatter rugs. Prepare some meals ahead of time and store them in the freezer, or purchase frozen prepared foods. You may be eligible for a temporary disabled parking permit, which can be obtained from your state department of motor vehicles.

You will need some assistance at first with household tasks like cleaning and shopping and with some personal tasks, like bathing. Depending on your medical condition, a visiting nurse or home health aide may be helpful.

You have a major role to play in the success of your surgery. Your active participation in a rehabilitation program is the key. Think of yourself as an athlete training to come back from an injury. The first several weeks require much effort. Several times a day, you will perform exercises your physical therapist has recommended to restore movement in the joint and strengthen the surrounding muscles (see Figure 13, page 42, and Figure 14, page 43). You can do many of these exercises while sitting or lying down. A physical therapist may come to your home or schedule regular appointments for the first few weeks. In addition to formal exercises, if you gradually increase the amount you walk and do normal tasks, your strength and stamina will improve.

You will need to use crutches or a walker for a

Possible complications of joint replacement

The success rate for knee and hip replacement is very high. However, complications can occur that shorten the life of an implant, and you may need to take certain precautions.

Infection. Your implant can become infected soon after surgery or years later. When it occurs later, it is almost always because infection elsewhere in the body has spread to the area. Seek immediate treatment if you have symptoms of an infection in the urinary tract or elsewhere, and inform all your doctors that you have a joint replacement.

Leg-length discrepancy. A difference in leg length occurs only rarely after knee replacement. But it happens frequently, at least temporarily, after hip replacement. Before surgery, one leg is often shorter than the other—or feels shorter because the joint has deteriorated. Your orthopedic surgeon chooses an implant and plans surgery so that your legs will be equal in length after healing. After

hip replacement, muscle weakness or spasm and swelling around the hip may temporarily cause an abnormal tilt to your pelvis and make you feel as though your legs are unequal in length. Stretching and strengthening exercises help restore your pelvis to its proper position. It may be several months before you can tell if the discrepancy is real and needs to be addressed with the use of a lift in one shoe. When the discrepancy is accompanied by pain, surgery can correct both problems.

Dislocation. In the weeks after a hip replacement, you'll need to take great care to keep from dislocating the implant before the surrounding tissues have healed enough to hold it in place. Even afterward, there is a chance of a painful dislocation. If your

hip dislocates, your doctor gives you a sedative while he or she manipulates the implant ball back into the socket. A hip that dislocates more than once usually requires additional surgery to make the joint more stable.

Loosening. A replacement joint can loosen because the cement never secured it properly or eventually wore out, or because the surrounding bone never grew into the implant to create a tight attachment. This may require a second surgery.

Bone loss. As a joint implant suffers wear and tear, loose particles can be released into the joint. As your immune system attacks these foreign particles, it can also attack surrounding bone, weakening it in a process called osteolysis. This, in turn, may loosen the bone's connection to the implant. Osteolysis is a major factor leading to the need for more surgery after hip and knee replacement.

period of time to keep weight off the implant. How long you will need to do this depends on different factors, including the type of implant. Most people can put a little weight on a cemented implant right away. An uncemented implant isn't secure until bone grows into it. You will probably be allowed to put only about half your weight on the joint for the first six weeks. With both types of implant, you should be able to walk without crutches or a walker by six weeks.

At that point, rehabilitation goals will shift toward restoring your ability to do normal activities, although you may still experience muscle pain and fatigue for several months as your tissues heal.

You should be able to function normally six months after the surgery. You can expect to have at least as much movement as you had before the operation, but with much less pain.

Guidelines for recovery from knee replacement

Ask your doctor and physical therapist how soon you can return to specific activities after knee replacement.

Driving. If your left knee was replaced, you may be able to drive a car with an automatic transmission as soon as you are not taking opioid medication and feel up to it. If the right knee was operated on, you will probably have to wait six to eight weeks.

Work. If you sit at a desk most of time while at your job, you can probably return to work after six to eight weeks. If your job requires you to stand, walk, or lift heavy objects, it may be three or four months before you can return.

Sex. The incisions and tissues in the front of the knee must be healed. This should take about six weeks. To avoid putting weight on your knees during sex, try a position that involves lying on your back or side or even sitting.

Sports. By eight weeks after surgery, you may be able to resume low-impact activities such as golfing, bowling, ballroom dancing, biking, swimming, or scuba diving. However, a knee implant may not hold up to high-impact activities that require lots of jumping, twisting, or repeated hard landings, such as running, soccer, basketball, volleyball, or contact sports. Ask your doctor whether a return to your favorite sport is realistic; if so, your physical therapist can help

---

Dos and don'ts after surgery

These tips can help ensure that your return to mobility goes smoothly.

Do eat right. Eating a healthy diet, including lots of fruits, vegetables, and whole grains, is important to promote proper tissue healing and restore muscle strength.

Do learn the signs of blood clots. Warning signs of a leg clot include increasing pain, tenderness, redness, or swelling in your knee and leg. Signs a clot has traveled to your lung include shortness of breath and chest pain that comes on suddenly with coughing. Call your doctor if you develop any of these signs.

Do look for signs of infection. These include persistent fever, shaking, chills, increasing redness or swelling of the knee, drainage from the surgical site, and increasing pain with both activity and rest.

Do exercise wisely. Performing the exercises your physical therapist recommends is crucial to restoring movement in your new joint and strengthening the surrounding muscles.

Don't soak your wound. Upon returning from the hospital, keep your wound dry until it has thoroughly sealed and dried.

Don't take risks that could cause you to fall. Use a cane, crutches, or a walker until you have improved your balance and strength. Be especially careful on stairs.

---

tailor your rehab program to prepare you for the safest return possible.

Guidelines for recovery from hip replacement

After hip replacement, talk to your doctor and physical therapist about activities that are encouraged or prohibited.

Car travel. Your physical therapist can provide instructions for getting in and out of the car and riding safely. Some vehicles are unacceptably high or low, forcing your hip into an unhealthy position. In some cars, sitting on a firm pillow can help you avoid over-flexing your hip. On long drives, stop and get out at least once an hour.

Driving. It usually takes about six weeks before you can drive a car with an automatic transmission and 12 weeks for a stick shift. You must be off any opioid pain medications, and you need to be able to put weight on your right leg (for an automatic transmission) or both legs (in the case of a manual transmission). You must also be able to brake without violating your hip precautions.

Sex. Wait until muscles and incisions have healed, which can take several weeks. You can resume sexual activity when the surgical wound is no longer painful and your doctor says it's okay. You may need to lie on your back or on the side that wasn't operated on. Avoid flexing your hips more than 90°, and don't raise your knees higher than your hips. Also, do not rotate your hips outward (either sitting or lying with knees wide apart).

Work. It may take three to six months before you can return to work. With a desk job, you can return sooner than if your job is more physically demanding. If you sit at a desk, your chair should have arms and be high enough to properly position your hips.

Sports. After a few months, you should be able to return to activities such as golf, biking (without steep hills), and ballroom or square dancing. Avoid activities that require jumping or heavy lifting, might jolt or stress your hip, or make it likely you might fall or have

something (or someone) bump into your hip. This means that tennis, volleyball, horseback riding, skating, contact sports, soccer, squash, and racquetball are usually not advisable.

Replacing other joints

Hips and knees are the most common joints replaced, but there are replacement options for other joints as well, such as shoulders, ankles, and fingers.

Shoulder replacement. Like the hip joint, the shoulder joint is a ball and socket. The ball at the top of the upper arm bone (humerus) fits into a socket in the shoulder blade (the glenoid cavity). A standard shoulder joint replacement involves inserting a long stem with a metal ball on the end into the humerus. A plastic cup replaces the socket. This provides pain relief and improved function for people who have osteoarthritis in the shoulder.

Shoulder replacement works best if you don't also have a damaged rotator cuff. The rotator cuff is the group of muscles and tendons that surround the shoulder joint and connect the humerus to the shoulder blade. The rotator cuff can weaken and tear over time. People with a torn rotator cuff are not helped

---

Figure 13: Exercises after knee replacement

Under the guidance of your physical therapist, you'll gradually be able to do the following exercises:

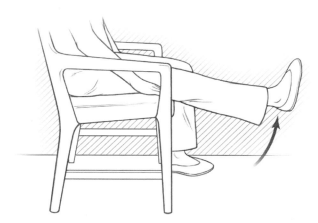

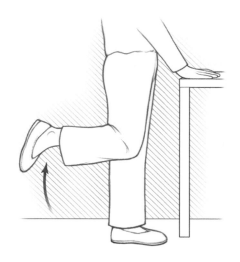

Sitting knee bends: Sit in a chair with a towel (not shown) under the operated knee. Straighten your knee as far as possible and hold for five seconds. Repeat 10 times. Gradually work up to 25 repetitions.

Standing knee bends: Hold on to a steady surface such as a table. Bend your operated knee back as far as you reasonably can. Hold for five seconds, then lower the leg to the floor. Repeat 10 times. Gradually work up to 25 repetitions.

Figure 14: Exercises after hip replacement

Check with your physical therapist to find out if you are ready to do the following exercises to strengthen your hip.

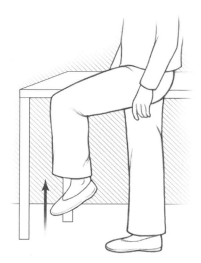

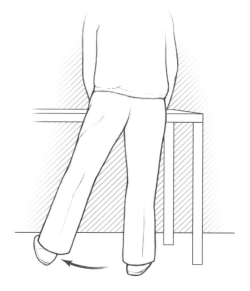

Standing knee raises: Standing with the aid of a walker or holding a stable surface, lift your thigh and bend your knee. Hold for five to 10 seconds. Repeat until your leg feels fatigued.

Hip abduction: Standing with your hand on a stable surface, lift your leg out to the side as far as you can and hold for five to 10 seconds. Keep your hip, knee, and foot pointing straight forward. Repeat until your leg feels fatigued.

with a standard shoulder replacement. This is because the muscles of the rotator cuff keep the ball centered in the socket. If the muscles are badly torn, the implant is likely to be unstable. To address this, surgeons can perform a reverse shoulder replacement. With this procedure, the two pieces of the implant are put in the opposite places from usual: the ball doesn't replace the ball at the top of the humerus, but rather it's inserted into the shoulder blade, while the socket is placed at the top of the humerus. This positioning allows the stronger deltoid muscle rather than the weaker rotator cuff to stabilize, power, and move the joint.

Rehabilitation after shoulder replacement surgery, whether standard or reverse, starts with some gentle stretching to allow the shoulder to heal for about six weeks before undertaking a more active exercise program.

Ankle replacement. An ankle implant is composed of metal and plastic and has two components. The top component is a plate that is inserted into the end of the shin bone (tibia). The bottom component replaces the bone at the top of the foot (talus).

Ankle replacement is best suited for people not likely to engage in high-impact activities like jogging or tennis that put pressure on the ankles. As with other types of joint replacement, you will work with a physical therapist after the surgery to regain strength and mobility in the joint.

Joint replacements in the hand. Replacing joints in the hand is challenging because of the smaller size of the joints and intricate bone structure of the hand. But advances in materials and techniques have made it a viable option.

Osteoarthritis is common in the joint at the base of the thumb (the first carpometacarpal, or CMC, joint), and there are several surgical options for this joint. A commonly used approach involves removing the bone at the base of the thumb (trapezium) and replacing it with a piece of tendon that is taken from the forearm and folded up like an accordion. This acts as a cushion among the remaining bones in the wrist. Another option is a total joint replacement, in which a prosthetic implant is used.

The middle joint of the finger (the proximal interphalangeal, or PIP, joint) can also be replaced with an implant made of metal, plastic, or pyrocarbon. ▼

Other types of arthritis

Osteoarthritis is only one of 100 types of arthritis, all of which can affect one or more joints. It's possible to have more than one type of arthritis at once, especially as you get older. For example, you may have osteoarthritis together with rheumatoid arthritis, gout, or pseudogout. Each type of arthritis has distinct causes and symptoms, but symptoms may be similar enough that different types can be confused with one another. It's important to get an accurate diagnosis, because treatment for each type of arthritis will be different. After osteoarthritis, the most common are rheumatoid arthritis and gout, which are discussed in this chapter. Some less common forms of arthritis are covered in Table 1, page 46.

Rheumatoid arthritis

Rheumatoid arthritis is a chronic autoimmune disease in which the body's immune system attacks healthy tissue, primarily the tissue lining the joints. This causes joint inflammation, a process marked by swelling, pain, redness, and stiffness. It affects an estimated 1.5 million American adults, and it is more common in women. It usually appears during middle age, but it may occur as early as a person's 20s and 30s.

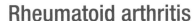

▶ Symptoms of rheumatoid arthritis

- Constant or recurring pain or tenderness in joints
- Stiffness and difficulty using or moving joints normally
- Swelling in and around multiple joints
- Warmth and redness in multiple joints
- Difficulty in performing daily tasks
- Arthritis in large and small joints in a more or less symmetrical pattern on both sides of the body
- Weight loss
- Fatigue
- Prolonged morning stiffness (more than 30 minutes)

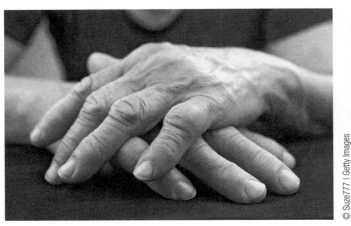

Gnarled, twisted fingers used to be common in people with rheumatoid arthritis. But disease-modifying drugs known as DMARDs now allow patients to reduce or prevent joint damage.

© Suze777 | Getty Images

Figure 15, page 45, illustrates joint changes that occur as a result of the chronic inflammation of rheumatoid arthritis.

Rheumatoid arthritis attacks multiple joints and is usually symmetrical, affecting joints on both sides of the body, particularly the finger joints, base of the thumbs, wrists, elbows, knees, ankles, or feet. It nearly always involves the wrists and the middle and large knuckles, but seldom the joints nearest the fingertips. At times, joint pain may be constant, even without movement. Morning stiffness that lasts for 30 minutes or longer is a hallmark of the disease.

The course of rheumatoid arthritis is unpredictable. Early on, the symptoms frequently abate or even disappear, only to flare up weeks or months later. Occasionally, complete remission occurs, usually within the first year. But for some people the process is destructive, ending in severe disability within a few years.

People with rheumatoid arthritis can develop eye conditions, including dry eye, which causes redness, burning, itching, reduced tearing, and sensitivity to light. Other complications of rheumatoid arthritis include respiratory, heart, and neurologic disorders.

In rare cases, the ligaments that tether the uppermost vertebrae (which support the skull) are damaged, allowing the vertebrae to slip out of alignment and pinch the spinal cord.

At advanced stages, rheumatoid arthritis can limit a person's ability to carry out normal daily activities such as dressing, bathing, and walking. However, medications help to slow the progression of rheumatoid arthritis and make a dramatic difference in the lives of many of those affected.

Causes of rheumatoid arthritis

Scientists don't know what causes rheumatoid arthritis, but they are investigating many hypotheses. The disorder runs in families, so it is likely that genes are an underlying factor in many cases. It has been theorized that hormones play some role in rheumatoid arthritis because the ailment affects more women than men. In addition, the symptoms often lessen during pregnancy and flare up again after delivery. Smoking cigarettes is known to increase the risk for rheumatoid arthritis. There also appears to be a link between rheumatoid arthritis and periodontal (gum) disease. Studies have found that people with rheumatoid arthritis are more likely to have gum disease than people without rheumatoid arthritis.

Diagnosing rheumatoid arthritis

Rheumatoid arthritis is generally diagnosed based on symptoms and a physical examination. Blood and imaging tests can help with the diagnosis. Most people with rheumatoid arthritis have an abnormal antibody called rheumatoid factor in their blood. Because this blood test is not definitive, other tests may also be needed. A test for anti-CCP measures the presence of an antibody strongly associated with rheumatoid arthritis. Tests for inflammation include measuring the erythrocyte sedimentation rate and measuring levels of C-reactive protein. People with osteoarthritis tend to have normal or negative results on all of these tests. (For details on these tests, see "Blood tests," page 13.)

Imaging tests (see page 14) may also help determine whether symptoms are caused by osteoarthritis or rheumatoid arthritis.

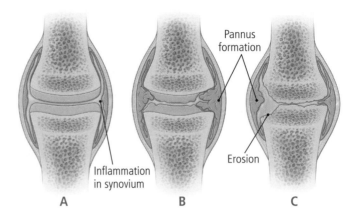

Figure 15: Joint changes in rheumatoid arthritis

A. Inflammation begins in the synovium.

B. The synovium begins to proliferate and forms pannus, a rough, grainy tissue that erodes cartilage.

C. Cells in the pannus release enzymes that eat into the cartilage, bone, and soft tissues. Nearby tendons and the joint capsule may become inflamed, causing pain, instability, deformity, weakness, loss of motion, and, occasionally, tendon rupture.

Treating rheumatoid arthritis

As with osteoarthritis, NSAIDs (see page 21) can help alleviate pain and inflammation. But unlike osteoarthritis, rheumatoid arthritis is also treatable with drugs that can actually slow the worsening of the disease. Therefore, early treatment is considered the best strategy to avoid joint damage. Drugs called disease-modifying antirheumatic drugs (DMARDs) alter the function of the immune system, which can slow the progression of rheumatoid arthritis. Because these medications can reduce or prevent joint damage and preserve joint function, they have become the first-line treatment and standard of care for most people with rheumatoid arthritis.

DMARDs, which work on the immune system in different ways, are divided into categories. Methotrexate and some other drugs produced through traditional means of making pharmaceutical drugs are called nonbiologic DMARDs. Drugs created through genetic engineering techniques are called biologic DMARDs. These drugs, which are delivered by injection or infusion, affect specific parts of the immune system. Newer drugs called janus kinase (JAK) inhibitors are in a separate drug category. They also affect the immune system and can be taken in pill form.

The first choice of a drug usually is the nonbiologic DMARD methotrexate (Folex, Rheumatrex, Trexall). Other nonbiologic DMARDs, which can be used alone or along with methotrexate, include hydroxychloroquine (Plaquenil), leflunomide (Arava), and sulfasalazine (Azulfidine). If these drugs don't work well enough, the other categories of drugs will be tried, alone or in various combinations.

Some people with rheumatoid arthritis require surgery to reconstruct or replace a damaged joint. Surgery is usually viewed as a last resort to reduce pain and improve function. Many procedures used to repair joints damaged by osteoarthritis are also used in rheumatoid arthritis. The most common surgical procedures for rheumatoid arthritis are arthroscopy, synovectomy (removal of the inflamed tissue that lines the joint), and arthroplasty (joint repair, including joint replacement).

Another Harvard Special Health Report, *Rheumatoid Arthritis: How to protect your joints, reduce pain, and improve mobility*, goes into much greater depth on all of these topics (see "Resources," page 52).

Table 1: Other types of arthritis

TYPE	SYMPTOMS	CAUSES	DIAGNOSTIC TESTS	TREATMENT
Ankylosing spondylitis Chronic, systemic inflammatory disease that often strikes people ages 20 to 40 and causes inflammation of the joints in the spine and pelvis. Eventually vertebrae in the spinal column may fuse.	Back pain and stiffness that develop gradually over weeks and persist for months Discomfort that is most noticeable in the morning, but improves with exercise	While the cause is unknown, people with this condition often have genes that make them more susceptible	X-rays, although it may take several years for the effects of the condition to show up on an image CT or MRI scan to detect inflammation in joints HLA-B27 (a genetic test)	NSAIDs Physical therapy Stretching exercises to extend the spine If symptoms do not improve, a DMARD or a biologic medication may be used
Bacterial arthritis Bacteria enter a joint or joints (most often a knee), causing arthritis. The germs may enter directly through a puncture wound or, more often, travel through the bloodstream from somewhere else in the body.	Joint inflammation, pain, and stiffness, typically in the knee, shoulder, ankle, or hip joints Fever and chills Rash (at isolated spots or all over the body)	Bacteria and other infectious organisms, including *Borrelia* (which causes Lyme disease), *Staphylococcus*, *Streptococcus*, gonorrhea, and tuberculosis	Removal of fluid from the affected joint for analysis Blood and urine tests	Antibiotics In some cases, surgery may be necessary
Enteropathic arthritis Develops in about 9% to 20% of people with ulcerative colitis or Crohn's disease, which are types of inflammatory bowel disease.	Arthritis in several joints, especially the knees, ankles, elbows, and wrists, and sometimes in the spine, hips, or shoulders Worsening of symptoms during flare-ups of inflammatory bowel disease	People with this form of arthritis have a hereditary disposition	Colonoscopy with biopsy	NSAIDs Corticosteroids DMARDs Anti-TNF or other biologic agents
Pseudogout Occurs when calcium crystals accumulate in the joints, especially the knee or wrist, though other joints may also be affected.	Severe pain, swelling, and stiffness around the joint(s) Fever, usually low-grade	Usually unknown Risk increases with age	X-ray to look for calcium deposits in the cartilage Removal of fluid from the affected joint to look for calcium crystals, inflammation, or infection Blood tests	NSAIDs, corticosteroids, or colchicine for pain and swelling Removal of fluid (aspiration) from the joint to relieve pressure

Continued on page 47

Gout

Gout is a form of arthritis with a very different cause than osteoarthritis. It develops in people with high levels of uric acid (a biological waste product) in their blood. When levels of uric acid get too high, it can settle in tissues throughout the body, particularly joints. From time to time, the uric acid forms needle-shaped crystals in the joint space. The body reacts to these crystals by launching an attack that causes inflammation, redness, and pain. This is called a gout attack. It usually lasts several days to a week and then subsides. Gout attacks often recur.

Gout usually affects a single joint at a time, most often the big toe, but sometimes a knee, ankle, wrist, foot, or finger instead. If gout persists for many years, uric acid crystals may collect in the joints or tendons and under the skin, forming whitish deposits known as tophi. Gout affects roughly six million Ameri-can men and two million American women. African American men are twice as likely as Caucasian men to be affected. Women rarely have gout until 10 or more years after menopause.

▶ **Symptoms of gout**

- Pain and swelling within a joint
- Often, an initial episode that occurs at night
- Shiny red or purple skin around the affected joint
- Extreme tenderness around the joint

Causes of gout

The cells of our bodies are constantly renewing themselves. Old cells die and are replaced with new ones. As dying cells break down, they release uric acid, which is a waste product of substances in cells called purines.

Table 1 *continued from page 46*

TYPE	SYMPTOMS	CAUSES	DIAGNOSTIC TESTS	TREATMENT
Psoriatic arthritis About 15% of people with psoriasis, a chronic skin disease, develop arthritis. It usually develops between the ages of 20 and 50.	Morning joint stiffness Joint pain and inflammation, particularly in the fingers, toes, or spine Pink or salmon scales on the scalp, knees, elbows, chest, or lower back Pitting of the fingernails or toenails	Unknown, although it probably arises from a combination of genetic and environmental factors	X-rays Blood tests Skin biopsy	NSAIDs If symptoms do not improve, a DMARD or biologic agent Corticosteroid injections may be used to control severe inflammation
Reactive arthritis Arthritis symptoms resulting from the immune system's response to an infection elsewhere in the body. Symptoms may develop weeks or months after the infection has cleared up and may flare suddenly, causing pain and stiffness, especially in the wrists, knees, ankles, and feet.	Fatigue, fever, muscle aches, and joint pain Low back pain radiating to the buttocks or thighs Discomfort aggravated by inactivity, eased by exercise Burning with urination Painful or irritated red eyes, blurry vision	May develop after infection with a sexually transmitted organism May be caused by gastrointestinal infection from bacteria such as *Salmonella, Shigella, Campylobacter,* or *Yersinia*	No specific diagnostic tests; review of earlier tests of urine, stool, or blood for evidence of prior infection	Antibiotics to treat the underlying infection NSAIDs or corticosteroids for pain and inflammation DMARDs in the case of prolonged attacks
Viral arthritis Viruses cause more cases of infectious arthritis than bacteria, but they are generally less serious.	Symptoms are similar to those of bacterial arthritis, but they usually abate as the virus is eliminated from the body	Viruses, including those that cause colds and respiratory infections Viruses causing serious illnesses such as AIDS and hepatitis C	Removal of fluid from the affected joint for analysis Blood and urine tests	No effective treatment for milder forms, as viruses don't respond to antibiotics Antiviral therapy for cases related to AIDS or hepatitis

The body removes uric acid through the gastrointestinal tract and kidneys. Much of it is expelled in urine.

Some people don't get rid of enough uric acid. If this happens, levels of uric acid can build up in the bloodstream. This condition is called hyperuricemia. In rare cases, the body produces too much uric acid, which also results in an excess of uric acid in blood. People with hyperuricemia can develop gout. But not everyone with high uric acid levels develops gout. The reasons for this are not well understood.

There are some known risk factors for gout. These include a family history of gout; overweight or obesity; high blood pressure; kidney disease; and use of certain medications, such as diuretics (used to treat high blood pressure, heart failure, and other conditions).

Certain foods and drinks can raise uric acid levels and may play a role in increasing the risk for gout or in triggering attacks in people who have gout. These include foods high in purines—especially organ meats (liver, kidney, and sweetbreads), red meat (beef, lamb, and pork), and some seafood (shellfish, anchovies, and sardines). Alcohol reduces the amount of uric acid removed by the kidneys, leaving more in circulation. Binge drinking can trigger gout attacks. Even moderate drinking can be problematic for some people with gout.

Diagnosing gout

Your doctor will ask you about your diet, your medication use, your alcohol consumption, and whether you have a family history of gout. During a physical exam, your doctor will inspect your inflamed joints and look for tophi, whitish deposits of uric acid under the skin. Your doctor may use a needle to withdraw a small fluid sample from your affected joint. This fluid will be examined under a microscope to determine whether uric acid crystals are present.

Treating gout

Gout is usually treated with a two-pronged strategy: the first goal is to ease joint pain and inflammation during attacks, while the second, longer-term goal is to prevent attacks in the future.

Treating an ongoing attack. NSAIDs often are prescribed to control pain and inflammation. A corticosteroid may be used if NSAIDs are ineffective or not tolerated. Oral colchicine (Mitigare, Colcrys) is another option, but this drug may cause unpleasant side effects (nausea, vomiting, cramps, diarrhea). Colchicine is effective for about 35% of gout sufferers.

Preventing future attacks. Long-term treatment of gout involves taking medication to lower levels of uric acid, an approach called urate-lowering therapy. Guidelines from the American College of Rheumatology recommend urate-lowering therapy for people who have been diagnosed with gout and have two or more attacks a year. Drug treatment is also recommended for anyone who has tophi and for people who have gout in addition to kidney disease or kidney stones.

The first choice is usually allopurinol (Aloprim, Zyloprim), which decreases your body's production of uric acid. It is available as a generic and therefore is the least expensive option. Another drug, febuxostat (Uloric) also cuts uric acid production. But because studies have linked febuxostat to a higher risk of dying from cardiovascular events compared with allopurinol, the FDA added a "black box" warning (the agency's strongest level of caution) to the package and also limited the approved use of the drug to cases where allopurinol is not effective or causes severe side effects.

Another option is Probenecid (Benemid, Probalan), which helps the kidneys eliminate uric acid, but people with kidney stones or kidney disease shouldn't take it. Lesinurad (Zurampic) also helps the kidneys remove uric acid. It's used together with allopurinol or febuxostat. Yet another option is pegloticase (Krystexxa), which is usually reserved for people who can't take or don't get relief from the other medications. This drug, which is given via intravenous infusion every two weeks, works by breaking down uric acid into a harmless chemical that's excreted in the urine.

You can also help prevent further attacks by avoiding diuretics (if your doctors agree), limiting your alcohol intake (no more than one drink a day for women and two for men), drinking plenty of water, and maintaining a healthy weight. Rather than try to keep track of which foods contain purines and how much, experts recommend following an overall healthy diet that emphasizes plant-based foods. ◗

Appendix: Drugs for treating osteoarthritis

Topical pain relievers

One of these, diclofenac, is available only by prescription as a gel, liquid, or patch; all three forms relieve mild to moderate joint pain and inflammation. The others, which are available over the counter, are moderately effective for mild pain. Topical pain relievers work best on joints close to the skin, such as those in the knees and hands. Do not use on broken or irritated skin or in combination with a heating pad or bandage.

GENERIC NAME (BRAND NAME)	ACTIVE INGREDIENT	HOW IT WORKS	POSSIBLE SIDE EFFECTS	COMMENTS
capsaicin-based creams (Capzasin, Zostrix, others)	Capsaicin, derived from cayenne peppers	Depletes substance P, believed to send pain messages to the brain	Temporary burning or stinging at the application site, which usually disappears in a few weeks of continuous use	Wash your hands thoroughly after use. Avoid contact with the eyes.
counterirritants (Eucalyptamint, Icy Hot, Therapeutic Mineral Ice, others)	Pungent oils derived from mint, wintergreen, eucalyptus, and other plants	Stimulate or irritate nerve endings to distract the brain's awareness of pain	Skin redness and irritation at application site	Many of these products have strong odors.
diclofenac (Flector Patch, Pennsaid, Voltaren Gel)	A nonsteroidal anti-inflammatory drug (NSAID)	Inhibits prostaglandins, hormone-like substances that contribute to pain and inflammation	Skin redness and irritation at application site	Do not use with oral NSAIDs. Long-term users should receive periodic blood tests to monitor liver function.
lidocaine patch (Lidoderm)	Lidocaine hydrochloride	Stops nerves from sending pain signals	Irritation, redness, swelling, numbness, changes in skin color at the application site	Lower-strength versions are available without a prescription. Higher-strength versions are by prescription only.
salicylates (ArthriCare, Aspercreme, Bengay, Flexall, Mobisyl, Sportscreme, others)	A type of NSAID derived from willow tree bark	Same as both diclofenac and counterirritants	Skin redness and irritation at application site	Do not use if you are allergic to aspirin or are taking blood thinners.

Oral pain relievers

Depending on your level of pain, an over-the-counter drug may be sufficient, or you may need to step up to a prescription drug.

GENERIC NAME (BRAND NAME)	USE	POSSIBLE SIDE EFFECTS	COMMENTS
▼ Over-the-counter products			
For mild to moderate pain. All of these medications, with the exception of acetaminophen, are NSAIDs and should be taken with food, milk, or an antacid to minimize stomach problems.			
acetaminophen (Tylenol, others)	Relieves pain	Nausea, vomiting, diarrhea, jaundice, rash, tiredness, weakness; less likely to cause gastric bleeding than other pain relievers	Drinking large amounts of alcohol during long-term therapy with acetaminophen may cause liver damage. Kidney damage also possible with long-term use.

Continued on page 50

GENERIC NAME (BRAND NAME)	USE	POSSIBLE SIDE EFFECTS	COMMENTS
aspirin (Bayer, Bufferin, others)	Reduce inflammation and relieve pain	Stomach pain, bleeding, ulcers; increased risk for heart attack and stroke with ibuprofen and naproxen	High doses may cause ringing in the ears. Before using, let your doctor know if you are on blood thinners or have liver or kidney problems.
ibuprofen* (Advil, Motrin, others)			Stronger and generally longer-lasting than aspirin.
naproxen* (Aleve)			Longer-lasting than ibuprofen.

*Ibuprofen and naproxen are available in higher doses by prescription only. Naproxen is also sold by prescription in combination with a medication to suppress stomach acid (either lansoprazole or esomeprazole), under the brand names Prevacid NapraPAC 500 and Vimovo.

▼ Prescription NSAIDs (nonsteroidal anti-inflammatory drugs)

For moderate pain. All NSAIDs should be taken with milk, food, or an antacid to reduce the likelihood of gastrointestinal distress.

GENERIC NAME (BRAND NAME)	USE	POSSIBLE SIDE EFFECTS	COMMENTS
diclofenac (Voltaren, others) **diflunisal** (Dolobid) **etodolac** (generic) **fenoprofen** (Nalfon, others) **flurbiprofen** (Ansaid, others) **indomethacin** (Indocin, others) **ketoprofen** (Orudis, others) **meclofenamate** (Meclomen, others) **mefenamic acid** (Ponstel) **mobic** (Meloxicam) **nabumetone** (Relafen) **oxaprozin** (Daypro) **piroxicam** (Feldene) **sulindac** (Clinoril) **tolmetin** (generic)	Reduce inflammation and relieve pain	Stomach pain or bleeding, ulcers, weight loss, nausea, vomiting, drowsiness, dizziness, fluid retention, heartburn, diarrhea, constipation, blurred vision, tinnitus, increased risk for heart attack and stroke	Rare allergic reactions; do not take if you are allergic to aspirin. High doses can cause ringing in the ears. People who take high doses for a long time should have periodic blood tests to check for bleeding and liver or kidney damage. May cause kidney damage in people who are dehydrated, or who already have a kidney problem or heart failure.
celecoxib (Celebrex)		Stomach upset, fluid retention; fewer gastrointestinal side effects than traditional NSAIDs, but a possible increased risk of heart attack or stroke	Same as above. In addition, do not take celecoxib if you are allergic to sulfonamide antibiotics, and talk with your doctor first if you have heart disease.

▼ Prescription opiates

Typically used only when other medications don't provide adequate relief. Because of the risk of addiction, these drugs should only be taken intermittently for short periods (a week or so).

GENERIC NAME (BRAND NAME)	USE	POSSIBLE SIDE EFFECTS	COMMENTS
codeine (usually generic, combined with other pain relievers such as acetaminophen, as in Tylenol No. 3)	Relieve pain	Constipation, dizziness, nausea, vomiting, sleepiness	Take with food or milk. Do not drive while taking this medication. May lead to physical or emotional dependence; do not take if you have a history of substance abuse.
hydrocodone (Vicodin, Lortab, Norco)		Constipation, dizziness, headaches, nausea, vomiting, sleepiness	Usually not considered as a first approach for chronic pain conditions. May lead to physical or emotional dependence; do not take if you have a history of substance abuse. Avoid alcohol if you're taking this drug.
oxycodone (Percocet, Oxycontin)		Constipation, dizziness, dry mouth, headaches, nausea, vomiting, sleepiness	
tramadol (Ultram)		Constipation, dizziness, headaches, nausea, vomiting, sleepiness	Do not use if you have a history of substance abuse or if you suffer from asthma, kidney problems, or liver problems. Avoid alcohol if you're taking this drug.

Continued on page 51

Medications injected into the joint

GENERIC NAME (BRAND NAME)	USE	POSSIBLE SIDE EFFECTS	COMMENTS
injectable corticosteroids (various); commonly called steroids	Relieve pain and suppress inflammation of osteoarthritis, as well as bursitis and tendinitis, which may accompany osteoarthritis	Tenderness, burning, or tingling at injection site; thinning of skin at injection site; joint infections; cartilage damage	Injected into joints, tendon sheaths, or bursae. Serious systemic side effects seldom occur. Although both oral and injected steroids are used for rheumatoid arthritis, only the injected form is used for osteoarthritis.
hyaluronate (Euflexxa, Hyalgan, Monivisc, Orthovisc, Supartz, Synvisc)	Treats arthritis of the knee	Irritation at the injection site, swelling, bruising, mild pain, stiffness, or warmth in or by the knee, back pain, muscle pain	Hyaluronate is a synthetic version of hyaluronic acid, a natural substance that lubricates joints. These injections are approved by the FDA only for knee osteoarthritis.

Resources

Organizations

American Academy of Orthopaedic Surgeons
9400 W. Higgins Road
Rosemont, IL 60018
847-823-7186
www.aaos.org

This nonprofit organization provides education and services for orthopedic surgeons and other health professionals. The website includes patient information and a doctor referral service.

American College of Rheumatology
2200 Lake Blvd. NE
Atlanta, GA 30319
404-633-3777
www.rheumatology.org

This professional organization of physicians, health professionals, and scientists engages in education, research, and advocacy to improve the care of people with arthritis and other rheumatic and musculoskeletal diseases. It also offers practical support to health care providers.

Arthritis Foundation
1355 Peachtree St. NE, 6th floor
Atlanta, GA 30309
404-872-7100
844-571-HELP (toll-free helpline)
www.arthritis.org

This nonprofit foundation sponsors public education programs and continuing education for professionals, raises money for research, and publishes patient information materials. Local chapters can advise about doctors and sponsor activities such as swimming and self-help classes.

National Institute of Arthritis and Musculoskeletal and Skin Diseases
National Institutes of Health
1 AMS Circle
Bethesda, MD 20892
877-226-4267 (toll-free)
www.niams.nih.gov

This federal agency distributes patient and professional education materials about arthritis and rheumatic diseases. It also refers people to other sources of information.

Harvard Special Health Reports

The following Special Health Reports and Online Guides from Harvard Medical School will give you more in-depth information about some of the topics addressed in this report. You can order them by going online to www.health.harvard.edu or by calling 877-649-9457 (toll-free).

All About Gout
Robert H. Shmerling, M.D., Medical Editor
(Harvard Medical School, 2018)

This online-only guide explores the causes and symptoms of the disease, prevention, treatments, and lifestyle changes that can help.

Better Balance: Simple exercises to improve stability and prevent falls
Suzanne Salamon, M.D., and Brad Manor, Ph.D., Medical Editors
With Michele Stanten, Fitness Consultant
(Harvard Medical School, 2017)

Stiff, sore joints hamper movement. If your ankles or knees are arthritic, it's hard to bend them, which affects your ability to balance and react when you trip. Often, people begin moving less, and muscles essential to balance grow weaker still. The safe, effective balance exercises in this report can help stop this cycle.

Healthy Hands: Strategies for strong, pain-free hands
Barry P. Simmons, M.D., and Joanne P. Bosch, P.T., C.H.T., Medical Editors
(Harvard Medical School, 2018)

This report covers many common and uncommon hand conditions that can cause pain and other symptoms. It also provides solutions, including exercise, medication, surgery, and more.

An Introduction to Tai Chi: A gentle exercise program for mental and physical well-being
Peter M. Wayne, Ph.D., Medical Editor
(Harvard Medical School, 2017)

Studies show that tai chi can help with everything from lowering blood pressure and managing depression to building strength and improving balance. This report lays out the benefits and helps you create your own tai chi practice, including three simple routines for beginners.

An Introduction to Yoga
Sat Bir Shingh Khalsa, Ph.D., and Lauren E. Elson, M.D., Medical Editors
(Harvard Medical School, 2016)

This report presents a basic yoga program that can help improve your strength, balance, and flexibility, while also promoting mindfulness and greater well-being.

The Joint Pain Relief Workout: Healing exercises for your shoulders, hips, knees, and ankles
Lauren E. Elson, M.D., Medical Editor
With Michele Stanten, Fitness Consultant
(Harvard Medical School, 2018)

Designed by knowledgeable exercise experts, these workouts are intended to strengthen the muscles that support your joints, increase flexibility, and improve range of motion. Done regularly, these exercises can ease pain, improve mobility, and help prevent further injury.

Knees and Hips: A troubleshooting guide to knee and hip pain
Scott David Martin, M.D., Medical Editor
(Harvard Medical School, 2018)

This report describes the most common knee and hip conditions, from osteoarthritis to bursitis, tendinitis, torn menisci, ruptured tendons, labral tears, hip fractures, and more. It highlights information about medical treatments and surgery, with special emphasis on joint replacement options.